PDQ[*] SERIES

---

[*]*PDQ* (Pretty Darned Quick)

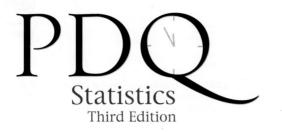

PDQ
Statistics
Third Edition

GEOFFREY R. NORMAN, PhD
Professor of Clinical Epidemiology and Biostatistics
McMaster University
Hamilton, Ontario

DAVID L. STREINER, PhD
Professor of Psychiatry
University of Toronto
Toronto, Ontario

2003
BC Decker Inc
Hamilton • London

People's Medical Publishing House
2 Enterprise Drive, Suite 509
Shelton, CT 06484
Tel: 203-402-0646
Fax: 203-402-0854
E-mail: info@pmph-usa.com

PMPH-USA

09 10 11 12 13/PMPH/9 8 7 6 5

ISBN: 978-1-55009-207-3

Printed in China by People's Medical Publishing House

Sales and Distribution

Canada
McGraw-Hill Ryerson
Education
Customer Care
300 Water St
Whitby, Ontario L1N 9B6
Canada
Tel: 1-800-565-5758
Fax: 1-800-463-5885
www.mcgrawhill.ca

Foreign Rights
John Scott & Company
International Publisher's
Agency
P.O. Box 878
Kimberton, PA 19442
USA
Tel: 610-827-1640
Fax: 610-827-1671

Japan
United Publishers Services
Limited
1-32-5 Higashi-Shinagawa
Shinagawa-ku, Tokyo
140-0002
Japan
Tel: 03-5479-7251
Fax: 03-5479-7307
Email: kakimoto@ups.co.jp

United Kingdom, Europe,
Middle East, Africa
McGraw Hill Education
Shoppenhangers Road
Maidenhead
Berkshire, SL6 2QL
England
Tel: 44-0-1628-502500
Fax: 44-0-1628-635895
www.mcgraw-hill.co.uk

Singapore, Thailand,
Philippines, Indonesia, Vietnam,
Pacific Rim, Korea
McGraw-Hill Education
60 Tuas Basin Link
Singapore 638775
Tel: 65-6863-1580
Fax: 65-6862-3354
www.mcgraw-hill.com.sg

Australia, New Zealand
Elsevier Australia
Tower 1, 475 Victoria Avenue
Chatswood NSW 2067
Australia
Tel: 0-9422-8553
Fax: 0-9422-8562
www.elsevier.com.au

Brazil
Tecmedd Importadora e
Distribuidora
de Livros Ltda.
Avenida Maurilio Biagi 2850
City Ribeirao, Rebeirao,
Preto SP
Brazil
CEP: 14021-000
Tel: 0800-992236
Fax: 16-3993-9000
Email:
tecmedd@tecmedd.com.br

India, Bangladesh, Pakistan,
Sri Lanka, Malaysia
CBS Publishers
4819/X1 Prahlad Street 24
Ansari Road, Darya,
New Delhi-110002
India
Tel: 91-11-23266861/67
Fax: 91-11-23266818
Email:cbspubs@vsnl.com

People's Republic of China
PMPH
Bldg 3, 3rd District
Fangqunyuan, Fangzhuang
Beijing 100078
P.R. China
Tel: 8610-67653342
Fax: 8610-67691034
www.pmph.com

This book is dedicated to the tens of thousands
of individuals who purchased copies of the first and
second editions, and to the many who wrote to tell
us how much they enjoyed the book. It is these people
who inspired us to write a third edition.
Thank you.

Preface to Third Edition

The second edition of PDQ *Statistics* came out 11 years after the first, and now the third edition appears on the scene only 5 years after the second. Has the pace of change in statistics grown so much that it's halved the time necessary for bringing out a new edition? Not really. The majority of what we've added has been around for a decade or three. What's changed is us. Now that all of the kids are grown and out of our homes (at least, we hope so), we have more time for pursuits other than dealing with minor and not-so-minor adolescent crises; things like carpentry (GRN), woodworking (DLS), traveling (both of us), and—when there's any time left over—learning some new statistical techniques. So, much of the new stuff (hierarchical and logistic regression, path analysis, and structural equation modeling) is what we've been playing with these last few years.

The other change is that both computer programs and journals have become more sophisticated, so it's not unusual to come across these techniques in clinical articles. Also, editors and grant review panels have (finally) become aware of the problems of missing data, so that topic has also been added to this edition.

What hasn't changed is the style. We've continued to keep equations to an absolute minimum (to stress concepts rather than math) and to assume that humor isn't antithetical to learning (and may in fact enhance it) and that people who get hung up on political correctness will have already heard about us and won't be reading this book. So if you feel you need humorless and politically correct dry math, return this book and get a refund. For the rest of you, enjoy!

G.R.N.
D.L.S.
January 2003

Contents

Introduction

Warning: This is not an introductory textbook in statistics. Introductory textbooks imply that you will go on to intermediate textbooks and then to advanced textbooks. As a result, introductory textbooks usually deal with only a few of the topics in the discipline. So if you want to apply your introductory knowledge of statistics to examining journals, most of the topics used by researchers won't have been covered.

Introductory textbooks have a couple of other problems. By and large, they are written by experts with the hope of enticing others to become experts, so they are written in the language of the discipline. Now it is certainly an important goal to understand the jargon; in most cases, once you get beyond the language, things get a bit simpler. But jargon can be an impediment to learning. Also, beginning textbooks usually are written on the assumption that the only way you can understand an area is to plunge up to your neck in the nitty-gritty details of equation-solving, theorem-proving, or number-juggling. At some level, that's probably legitimate. We're not sure we'd like a surgeon who hasn't actually removed an appendix to perform this procedure, even though he or she has a good conceptual grasp of the relevant anatomy and operating procedures. But we are going to assume that all that work is not necessary to understand an area, so we'll try to minimize the use of algebra, calculus, and calculations, and we'll use ordinary English as much as possible.

The intent of this book is to help you through the results section of a research article where the numbers are actually crunched, and little asterisks or "p < .05" values appear as if by magic in the margins, to the apparent delight of the authors. We think that by reading this book, you won't actually be able to do any statistics (actually, with computers on every street corner, no one—doctor, lawyer, beggarman, or statistician—should have to do statistics), but you will understand what researchers are doing and may even be able to tell when they're doing it wrong. There is an old joke about the three little French boys, ages 4, 5, and 6, who saw a man and a woman naked on a bed in a basement apartment. They said:

Four-Year-Old-Boy: Look at that man and that woman in there! They are wrestling!
Five-Year-Old-Boy: No silly, they are making love.
Six-Year-Old-Boy: Yes, and very poorly, too!

The 4-year-old boy knew nothing of lovemaking. The 5-year-old boy had achieved a conceptual understanding, and the 6-year-old boy understood lovemaking sufficiently well, presumably without actually having done it, to be a critical observer. The challenge of this book will be to turn you into a 6-year-old statistician. So, we will not take the "Introductory Textbook" approach in this book. Instead, we will expose you to nearly every kind of statistical method you are likely to encounter in your reading. Our aim is to help you understand what is going on with a particular approach to analysis, and furthermore, we hope you will understand enough to recognize when the author is using a method incorrectly. Along the way, you can leave the calculator on the back shelf, because it won't be needed.

One cautionary note: It would be nice if we could hand you an encyclopedia of statistical tests so you could just turn to page whatever and read about the particular test of interest. But statistics isn't quite like that. Like most things in science, it is built up logically on fundamental principles and evolves gradually to greater complexity. To gain some appreciation of the underlying concepts, it probably behooves you to start at the beginning and read to the end of the book at least once.

We hope that as a result of reading this book you will find the results section of journal articles a little less obscure and intimidating and thereby become a more critical consumer of the literature. It would not be surprising if you emerged with a certain degree of skepticism as a result of your reading. However, it would be unfortunate if you ended up dismissing out of hand any research advanced statistical methods simply because of your knowledge of the potential pitfalls. Keep in mind that the objective of all statistical analyses is to reveal underlying systematic variation in a set of data, either as a result of some experimental manipulation or from the effect of other measured variables. The strategy, which forms the basis of all statistical tests, is a comparison between an observed effect or difference and the anticipated results of random variation. Like a good stereo receiver, statistical analysis is designed to pluck a faint signal out of a sea of noise.

Unfortunately, also like a modern stereo receiver, the statistical methods are contained in black boxes like SPSS and SAS; prominent stickers proclaim that they should be opened by qualified personnel only so that it is nearly impossible to understand the detailed workings of a MANOVA, factor analysis, or logistic regression program. Finally, to complete the analogy, these boxes of software seem replete with endless switches and dials in the form of obscure tests or optional approaches, which may be selected to execute the programs and report the results.

It is understandable that many people in the research community react toward new statistical methods in the same way that they might react to other new technology; either they embrace the techniques openly and uncritically, or they reject any examples out of hand. Neither response is appropriate. These methods, available now through the development of sophisticated computer hardware and software, have made an enormous contribution to research in the social and health sciences. Nevertheless, they can be used appropriately or they can be abused, and the challenge that faces the reader is to decide whether a particular example is one or the other.

Let us say ahead of time what statistics cannot do to help place this book in an appropriate context.

The probability or "p" level associated with any test of significance is only a statement of the likelihood that an observed difference could have arisen by chance. Of itself, it says nothing about the size or importance of an effect. Because probability level is so closely related to sample size, small effects in large studies can achieve impressive levels of significance. Conversely, studies involving small numbers of subjects may have too little power to detect even fairly large effects.

No statistical method can effectively deal with the systematic biases that may result from a poorly designed study. For example, statistical techniques may be used to adjust for initial differences between two groups, but there is no way to ensure that this adjustment compensates exactly for the effect of these differences on the results of the study. Similarly, no statistical analysis can compensate for low response rates or high dropouts from a study. We can demonstrate ad nauseam that the subjects who dropped out had the same age, sex, marital status, education, and income as those who stayed in, but this is no guarantee that they would have been comparable to the variables that were measured in the study. The mere fact that they dropped out implies that they were different on at least one dimension, namely the inclination to remain in the study. Finally, no measure of association derived from natural variation in a set of variables, however strong, can establish with certainty that one variable caused another. To provide you with some tools to sort out the different experimental designs, we have included a critical review of the strengths and weaknesses of several designs in Chapter 18.

Finally, even after you are satisfied that a study was conducted with the appropriate attention to experimental design and statistical analysis and that the results are important, there remains one further analysis that you, the reader, can conduct. Whether you are a researcher or clinician, you must examine whether the results are applicable to the people with whom you deal. Are the people studied in the research paper sufficiently similar to your patients that the effects or associations are likely to be similar? For example, treatments that have significant effects when applied to severely ill patients in a university teaching hospital may be ineffective when used to treat patients with the same, albeit milder, form of the disease that is encountered in a general practice. Similarly, psychological tests developed on university undergraduates may yield very different results when applied to a middle-aged general population. The judgment as to the applicability

---

*Convoluted Reasoning or Antiintellectual Pomposity
†Postman N, Weingartner C. Teaching as a subversive activity. New York: Dell; 1987.

of the research results to your setting rests primarily on the exercise of common sense and reasoning, nothing more.

One last word about the intent of this book. Although we would like think that a good dose of common sense and an understanding of the concepts of statistics will enable you to examine the literature critically, we're going to hedge our bets a bit. Throughout the book we highlight particular areas where researchers frequently misuse or misinterpret statistical tests. These are labeled as "C.R.A.P.* Detectors," with apologies to Ernest Hemingway†, and are intended to provide particular guides for you to use in reviewing any study. In applying your new knowledge, don't be intimidated by all the tables of numbers and hifalutin talk. Always keep in mind the advice of Winifred Castle, a British statistician, who wrote that "We researchers use statistics the way a drunkard uses a lamp post, more for support than illumination." Finally, we hope that you enjoy the book!

G.R.N
D.L.S.
May 1986

Part One

Variables and Descriptive Statistics

Names and Numbers:
Types of Variables

There are four types of variables. *Nominal* and *ordinal* variables consist of counts in categories and are analyzed using "nonparametric" statistics. *Interval* and *ratio* variables consist of actual quantitative measurements and are analyzed using "parametric" statistics.

S*tatistics provide a way* of dealing with numbers. Before leaping headlong into statistical tests, it is necessary to get an idea of how these numbers come about, what they represent, and the various forms they can take.

Let's begin by examining a simple experiment. Suppose an investigator has a hunch that clam juice is an effective treatment for the misery of psoriasis. He assembles a group of patients, randomizes them to a treatment and control group, and gives clam juice to the treatment group and something that looks, smells, and tastes like clam juice (but isn't) to the control group. After a few weeks, he measures the extent of psoriasis on the patients, perhaps by estimating the percent of body involvement or by looking at the change in size of a particular lesion. He then does some number crunching to determine if clam juice is as good a treatment as he hopes it is.

Let's have a closer look at the data from this experiment. To begin with, there are at least two variables. A definition of the term **variable** is a little hard to come up with, but basically it relates to anything that is measured or manipulated in a study. The most obvious variable in this experiment is the measurement of the extent of psoriasis. It is evident that this is something that can be measured. A less obvious variable is the nature of treatment—drug or placebo. Although it is less evident how you might convert this to a number, it is still clearly something that is varied in the course of the experiment.

A few more definitions are in order. Statisticians frequently speak of independent and dependent variables. In an experiment, the **independent variables** are those that are varied by and under the control of the experimenter; the **dependent variables** are those that respond to experimental manipulation. In the current example, the independent variable is the type of therapy—clam juice or placebo—and the dependent variable is the size of lesions or body involvement. Although in this example the identification of independent and dependent variables is straightforward, the distinction is not always so obvious. Frequently, researchers must rely on natural variation in both types of variables and look for a relationship between the two. For example, if an investigator was looking for a relationship between smoking and lung cancer, an ethics committee would probably take a dim view of ordering 1,000 children to smoke a pack of cigarettes a day for 20 years. Instead, the investigator must look for a relationship between smoking and lung cancer in the general adult population and must assume that smoking is the independent variable and that lung cancer is the dependent variable; that is, the extent of lung cancer depends on variations in smoking.

There are other ways of defining types of variables that turn out to be essential in determining the ways the numbers will be analyzed. Variables are frequently classified as **nominal**, **ordinal**, **interval**, or **ratio** (Figure 1-1). A **nominal variable** is simply a *named* category. Our clam juice versus placebo is one such variable, as is the sex of the patient, or the diagnosis given to a group of patients.

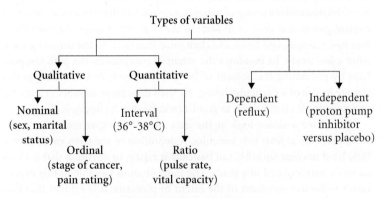

Figure 1-1 Types of variables.

An **ordinal variable** is a set of *ordered* categories. A common example in the medical literature is the subjective judgment of disease staging in cancer, using categories such as stage 1, 2, or 3. Although we can safely say that stage 2 is worse than stage 1 but better than stage 3, we don't really know by how much.

The other kinds of variables consist of actual measurements of individuals, such as height, weight, blood pressure, or serum electrolytes. Statisticians distinguish between **interval variables,** in which the interval between measurements is meaningful (for example, 32° to 38°C), and **ratio variables,** in which the ratio of the numbers has some meaning. Having made this distinction, they then analyze them all the same anyway. The important distinction is that these variables are measured *quantities*, unlike nominal and ordinal variables, which are *qualitative* in nature.

So where does the classification lead us? The important distinction is between the nominal and ordinal variables on one hand and the interval and ratio variables on the other. It makes no sense to speak of the average value of a nominal or ordinal variable—the average sex of a sample of patients or, strictly speaking, the average disability expressed on an ordinal scale. However, it is sensible to speak of the average blood pressure or average height of a sample of patients. For nominal variables, all we can deal with is the number of patients in each category. Statistical methods applied to these two broad classes of data are different. For measured variables, it is generally assumed that the data follow a bell curve and that the statistics focus on the center and width of the curve. These are the so-called **parametric statistics.** By contrast, nominal and ordinal data consist of counts of people or things in different categories, and a different class of statistics, called **nonparametric statistics** (obviously!), is used in dealing with these data.

C.R.A.P. DETECTORS

Example 1-1

To examine a program for educating health professionals in a sports injury clinic about the importance of keeping detailed medical records, a researcher does a controlled trial in which the *dependent* variable is the range of motion of injured joints, which is classified as (a) worse, (b) same, or (c) better, and the *independent* variable is (a) program or (b) no program.

Question. What kind of variables are these—nominal or ordinal? Are they appropriate?

Answer. The independent variable is *nominal*, and the dependent variable, as stated, is *ordinal*. However, there are two problems with the choice. First, detailed medical records may be a good thing and may even save some lives somewhere. But range of motion is unlikely to be sensitive to changes in recording behavior. A better choice would be some rating of the quality of records. Second, range of motion is a nice ratio variable. To shove it into three ordinal categories is just throwing away information.

C.R.A.P. Detector I-1

Dependent variables should be sensible. Ideally, they should be clinically important and related to the independent variable.

C.R.A.P. Detector I-2

In general, the amount of information increases as one goes from nominal to ratio variables. Classifying good ratio measures into large categories is akin to throwing away data.

2

Describing Data

A key concept in statistics is the use of a frequency distribution to reflect the probability of the occurrence of an event. The distribution can be characterized by measures of the average—mean, median, and mode—and measures of dispersion—range and standard deviation.

Once a researcher has completed a study, he or she is faced with some major challenges: to analyze the data in order to publish, to add a line to the CV, to get promoted or tenured, to get more research grants, and to analyze more data.

There are two distinct steps in the process of analyzing data. The first step is to describe the data by using standard methods to determine the average value, the range of data around the average, and other characteristics. The objective of **descriptive statistics** is to communicate the results without attempting to generalize beyond the sample of individuals to any other group. This is an important first step in any analysis. For a reader to understand the basis for the conclusions of any study, an idea of what the data look like is necessary.

The second step in some, but not all, studies is to infer the likelihood that the observed results can be generalized to other samples of individuals. If we want to show that clam juice is an effective treatment for psoriasis, or that intelligence (IQ) is related to subsequent performance, we are attempting to make a general statement that goes beyond the particular individuals we have studied. The rub is that differences between groups can rarely be attributed simply to the experimental intervention; some people in the clam juice group may get worse, and some people in the placebo group may get better. The goal of **inferential statistics** is to determine the likelihood that these differences could have occurred by chance as a result of the combined effects of unforeseen variables not under the direct control of the experimenter. It is here the statistical heavy artillery is brought to bear. As a result, most damage to readers of journals is inflicted by inferential statistics. Most of this book is devoted to the methods of statistical inference. However, a good idea of what the data look like is a necessary prerequisite for complex statistical analysis, both for the experimenter and the reader, so let's start there.

FREQUENCIES AND DISTRIBUTIONS

Whether a study involves 10 or 10,000 subjects, the researcher eventually ends up with a collection of numbers, often glorified by names such as "data set" or "database." In the case of nominal or ordinal variables, the numbers are an indicator of the category to which each subject belongs (for example, the sex, the religion, or the diagnosis of each subject). For interval and ratio variables, the researchers will have the actual numerical value of the variable for each subject—the subject's height, blood pressure, pulse rate, or number of cigarettes smoked. There is a subtle difference among these latter variables, by the way, even though all are ratio variables. Things like height and blood pressure are **continuous variables**; they can be measured to as many decimal places as the measuring instrument allows. By contrast, although the average American family has 2.1 children, no one has ever found a family with one-tenth of a child, making counts such as these **discrete variables**.

In either case, these numbers are distributed in some manner among the various categories or throughout the various possible values. If you plotted the numbers, you would end up with **distributions** similar to those shown in Figures 2-1 and 2-2.

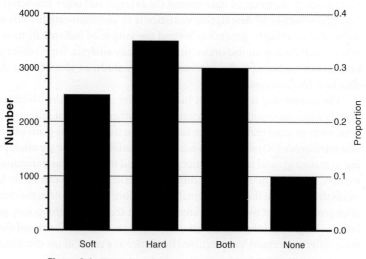

Figure 2-1 Distribution of ice cream preferences in 10,000 children.

Note that there are a couple of things that can be done to make these figures more understandable. If we divide the numbers in each category by the total number of people studied, we are then displaying the proportion of the total sample in each category, as shown on the right side of each graph. Some manipulations can be performed on these proportions. For example, to find the probability in Figure 2-2 that one of our folks is 69 or 70 years old, we must add up the probabilities in these 2-year categories. We can also address questions such as "What is the probability that a senior citizen is more than 71 years of age?" by adding the categories above age 71 years.

The basic notion is that we can view the original distribution of numbers as an expression of the probability that any individual chosen at random from the original sample may fall in a particular category or within a range of categories. This transformation from an original frequency distribution to a distribution of probability is a recurrent and fundamental notion in statistics.

Although a frequency distribution is a convenient way to summarize data, it has certain disadvantages. It is difficult to compare two distributions derived from different samples because the information is buried in the number of responses in each category. It's also tedious to draw graphs and a lot easier to get the computer to blurt out a series of numbers. As a result,

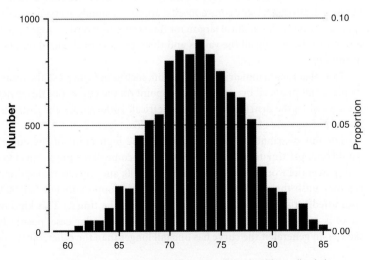

Figure 2-2 Age distribution of 10,000 entrants in senior citizen roller derby.

some way to summarize the information is necessary. The conventional approach is to develop standard methods that describe where the center of the distribution lies and how wide the distribution is.

MEASURES OF THE MIDDLE: MEANS, MEDIANS, AND MODES

For nominal data, there is no ordering implied in the various categories; we can't say that a preference for hard ice cream is, in any sense, better than a hatred of all ice cream. The best we can do is to indicate which category was most frequently reported; that is, in our ice cream study, "hard" was indicated most often. This value is called the **modal value** of the distribution. The modal value can be determined for all types of variables. For example, in Figure 2-2, the modal value is 73.

When we turn to ordinal variables, we see now an explicit or implied ordering to the categories of response. However, we don't know the spacing between categories. In particular, we cannot assume that there is an equal interval between categories, so any determination of an average that uses some measure of distance between categories is not legitimate. However, unlike with nominal variables, we do know that one category is higher or lower than another. For example, if we are talking about a rating of patient disability, it would be legitimate to ask the degree of disability of the average patient. So if we were to rank order 100 patients, with the "no disability" patients at the bottom and the "total disability" patients at the top, where would the dividing line between patient 50 and patient 51 lie? This value, with half the subjects below and half above, is called the **median value**.

For interval and ratio variables, we can use median and modal values, but we can also use a more commonsense approach, simply averaging all the values. The *mean* is statistical jargon for this straightforward average, which is obtained by adding all the values and then dividing by the total number of subjects.

Note that for a symmetrical distribution, such as in Figure 2-2, the mean, median, and mode all occur at the same point on the curve. But this is not the case when the distribution is asymmetrical. For example, the distribution of the income of physicians might look like Figure 2-3.

For this distribution, the *modal* value (the high point of the curve) would be approximately $50,000; the *median* income of the physician at the 50th percentile would be approximately $60,000; and the few rich specialists may push the *mean* or average income up to approximately $70,000. (Admittedly, these numbers are woefully behind the times.) This kind of curve is called a "skewed" distribution; in this particular case, positively skewed. In general, if the curve has one tail longer than the other, the mean

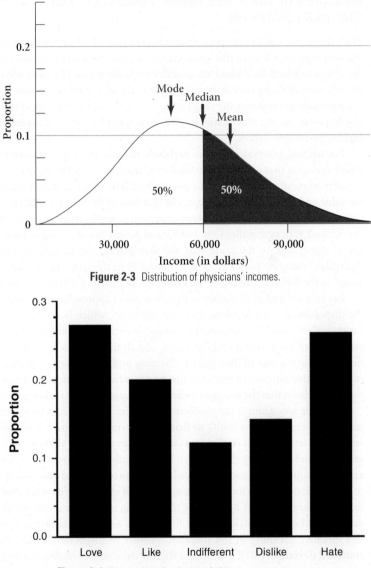

Figure 2-3 Distribution of physicians' incomes.

Figure 2-4 Distribution of attitudes of 100 teenagers to parents.

is always toward the long tail, the mode is nearer the short tail, and the median is somewhere between the two.

As a final wrinkle, in some data, there may be two or more high points in the distribution, such as in Figure 2-4. In this case, the distribution has two modes, love and hate, and is called "bimodal."

MEASURES OF VARIATION: RANGE, PERCENTILE, AND STANDARD DEVIATION

The various ways of determining an average provide a first step in developing summary measures of distributions, but we also need some measure of the extent to which individual values differ from the mean. The most obvious measure of dispersion is the **range**. For nominal variables, because the categories are not ordered, the range is the number of categories with at least one response. For the other variables, the range is the difference between the highest and lowest values.

For ordinal, interval, and ratio variables, there is another way to think about variation that is a natural extension of the concept of the median. As you should recall, the median is the point where 50% of the sample is below the value and 50% is above the value. The locations of the 0th and 100th percentiles would define the range. More commonly, people define the value of the 5th and 95th percentiles (5% and 95% of people below) as some measure of dispersion. In the same vein, the distribution can be divided into "quartiles," using cutpoints at 25%, 50%, and 75%; then, the "interquartile range" is the difference between the values of the 25th and 75th percentiles.

For interval and ratio variables, there is another approach to measuring the dispersion of individual values about the mean, which bears the name "average deviation." To compute the average deviation, calculate the difference between each datum and the mean, add all the differences, and then divide by the number of data points. The only problem is that there are as many negative differences from the mean as positive differences, and a little algebra shows that the average deviation calculated this way is always zero.

A simple way around the problem of negative differences is to square each term (multiply it by itself) so that all the terms are positive. You then would have terms such as (individual value − mean value)^2. If all these terms are added and the total is then divided by the number of terms, the result is an average squared deviation and is called a **variance**. Well and good, except that the variances are no longer in the same unit of measurement as the original data. For example, if height were measured in inches, the units of variance would be square inches. So the final step is to take the square root of this quantity, resulting in the standard measure of dispersion, called the **standard deviation** (SD). The SD is a slightly devious way of determining, on the average, how much the individual values differ from the mean. The smaller the SD (or s), the less each score varies from the mean. The larger the spread of scores, the larger the SD becomes. Algebraically, the formula looks like this:

$$SD = \sqrt{\frac{\text{sum of (individual value} - \text{mean value)}^2}{\text{number of values}}}$$

NORMAL DISTRIBUTION

Because much of what we will discuss in subsequent sections is based on the normal distribution, it's probably worthwhile to spend a little more time exploring this magical distribution.

It has been observed that the natural variation of many variables tends to follow a bell-shaped distribution, with most values clustered symmetrically near the mean and with a few values falling in the tails. The shape of this bell curve can be expressed mathematically in terms of the two statistical concepts we have discussed—the mean and the SD. In other words, if you know the mean and SD of your data, and if you are justified in assuming that the data follow a normal distribution, then you can tell precisely the shape of the curve by plugging the mean and SD into the formula for the normal curve.

If you look at the calculated curve superimposed on your mean and SD, you would see something like Figure 2-5.

Of the values, 68% fall within one SD of the mean, 95.5% fall within two SDs, and 2.3% fall in each tail. This is true for every normal distribution, not just this curve, and comes from the theoretical shape of the curve. This is a good thing because our original figures, such as those in Figure 2-2, don't really give much of an idea of what is happening on the tails. But we can use all the data to get a good estimate of the mean and SD, and then draw a nice smooth curve through it.

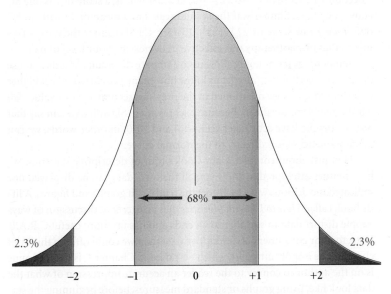

Figure 2-5 The normal distribution (bell-shaped curve).

STANDARD SCORES

Realizing that you've finished almost two chapters of a statistics book, you celebrate by taking a jog around the park. Not realizing how distracting statistics can be, you don't see the hole in the path, you twist your ankle, and you end up in the physiotherapy department. At the start of therapy, one therapist has you rate your pain on a 10-point scale, and you give it a score of 7. After 2 weeks, a different physiotherapist comes into the picture; she has you rate your pain on a different scale, and your score is 22. Have you gotten better, gotten worse, or stayed the same? It's hard to tell in this case because the scales obviously have different means, SDs, ranges, and so forth. Wouldn't it be nice if there were some way of expressing these scores along some common scale? Yes, it would, and it should come as no surprise to you that that's what we'll discuss now.

What we can do is change the raw scores (7 for the first scale and 22 for the second scale) into SD units; that is, we would say that the score is so many SDs above or below the mean, which are called standard scores or *z scores*. We do this by first determining how far above or below the mean the raw score is and then dividing that number by the SD, as follows:

$$\text{standard score } (z) = \frac{(\text{raw score} - \text{mean})}{\text{SD}}$$

So, if the mean of the first scale is 5 with an SD of 2, then a raw score of 7 becomes a z score of $(7 - 5)/2 = 1.0$; in other words, a score of 7 is one SD above the mean. Similarly, if the second scale has a mean of 15 with an SD of 5, then a raw score of 22 is $(22 - 15)/5 = 1.4$ SDs above the mean. This means that physiotherapy was effective in decreasing your level of pain.

Standard scores not only allow us to compare the results of tests that use different scales but they also let us know how many people would get higher or lower scores. As we mentioned in the previous section, 68% of values fall within one SD of the mean. Because z scores are in SD units, we can say that 68% of people have scores between -1.0 and $+1.0$; in other words, we can relate standard scores directly to the normal curve.

That just about completes our Cook's tour of descriptive statistics. We have neither attempted to show you all the ways data can be displayed nor indicated the devious ways to distort the truth with graphs and figures. A little book called *How to Lie with Statistics*[1] has an excellent discussion of ways people distort data to suit their own ends and has far more useful C.R.A.P. Detectors for consumers of descriptive data than we could offer in this brief chapter. The important point, which we raised in Chapter 1, is that the onus is on the author to convey to the reader an accurate impression of what the data look like, using graphs or standard measures, before beginning the statistical shenanigans. Any paper that doesn't do this should be viewed from the outset with considerable suspicion.

---

[1]Huff D. *How to lie with statistics.* New York: WW Norton; 1954.

Part Two

Parametric Statistics

3

Statistical Inference

Statistical Inference is the process of inferring features of the population from observations of a sample. The analysis addresses the question of the likelihood that an observed difference could have arisen by chance. The z test is the simplest example of a statistical test, and it examines the difference between a sample and a population when the variable is a measured quantity.

The story goes that one day Isaac Newton was slacking off in an apple orchard when an apple fell on his head, after which he invented the law of gravitation. It's a safe bet that Newton's goal wasn't to describe the motion of apples falling off trees—they usually don't hand out the Nobel Prize for things like that. Rather, he was attempting (successfully, as it turns out) to formulate a general rule based on his observations of specific instances.

Forgive a moment's pomposity, but that is really what science is all about: deriving general rules that describe a large class of events, based on observation and experiment of a limited subset of this class. There are at least two issues in this generalization. The first issue is that if the scientist wishes to have confidence in a generalization, he or she must be sure that the people or things chosen to study are representative of the class the scientist wants to describe. This notion leads to the fundamental role of random sampling in the design of experiments. The second issue is that there is always some experimental error associated with the process of measurement; when determining the value of some property of interest, the scientist must also provide a reasonable estimate of the likely error associated with the determination.

SAMPLES AND POPULATIONS

In Chapter 2, we discussed ways of describing data derived from a sample of people or things, called "descriptive statistics." When you get the poor folks to imbibe gallons of clam juice, your hope as an experimenter is to infer some general rule about the effects of clam juice on patients with psoriasis that holds true for more people than the people who actually were involved in the study. In statistical jargon, you want to make inferences about the **population,** based on the sample you have studied.

The statistical population has little to do with our everyday notion of population unless we're talking about census data or Gallup polls. The experimenter's population is the group of people about whom he or she wishes to make generalizations (eg, patients with psoriasis). In the best of all possible worlds, the experimenter should sample randomly from this population. In point of fact, this utopia can never be realized, if for no other reason than that any experimenter who doesn't have a free pass on the airlines (the exceptions are the scientists who do large multicenter multinational trials—they do seem to have free passes) is usually constrained by geography to a particular area of the country, but it's often safe to assume that American psoriasis is the same as British psoriasis. Still, in the end, it's up to the reader to judge the extent to which the results are generally applicable.

Despite the fact that no one ever really did random *sampling*, there is another randomizing process that everyone should do whenever they can—random *allocation*. Once you have your sample of folks together, by whatever means, if you now want to prove that your magic potion works, you have to form two groups: one that will get the potion and another that won't. To ensure that whatever differences measured at the end of the study really are due to something you did and not to self-selection, bias, or some other nasty effect, you should assign the individuals to get your potion or something else by using a coin flip or some other randomization device. This is called **random allocation**, and this is what "randomized" actually refers to in "randomized controlled trial." It is an essential ingredient in design (see Chapter 21) and is used as a way to ensure that you can be certain that the differences were caused by the treatment and not by something else.

STANDARD ERRORS

The second major issue arising from the game of statistical inference is that every measurement has some associated error that takes two forms: systematic error and random error. An example will clarify this. Suppose, for some obscure reason, we want to determine the height of 14-year-old boys in the United States. That's our population, but no agency will fund us to measure all 14-year-old boys in the country, so we settle for some samples of boys. For example, we randomly sample from 10 schools that were, in turn, randomly sampled throughout New York. Let's look at how our calculated mean height may differ from the true value, namely, that number obtained by measuring every boy in the United States and then averaging the results.

The idea of **systematic error** is fairly easy. If the ruler used is an inch short or if the schools have many northern Europeans, then regardless of how large a sample is or how many times we do the study, our results would always differ from the true value in a systematic way.

The notion of **random error** is a bit trickier but is fundamental to statistical inference. As an educated guess, the mean height of 14-year-olds is probably approximately 5 feet 8 inches, with a standard deviation (SD) of approximately 4 inches. This means that every time the experiment is performed, the results will differ depending on the specific kids who are sampled. This variation in the calculated mean, caused by individual measurements scattered around the true mean value, is called "random error." Actually, statistics are lousy at dealing with systematic error but awfully good at determining the effect of random error.

To illustrate, if we grabbed a few kids off the street, the chances are good that some of them might be very short or very tall, so our calculated mean may be far from the truth. Conversely, if we used thousands of kids, as long as they were sampled at random, their mean height value should fall close to the true population mean. As it turns out, the mean values determined from repeated samples of a particular size are distributed near the true mean in a bell-shaped curve with an SD equal to the original SD divided by the square root of the sample size. This new SD, describing the distribution of *mean* values, is called the **standard error** (SE) **of the mean** and is found as follows:

$$SE = \frac{SD}{\sqrt{sample\ size}}$$

Figure 3-1 illustrates how the SE is related to the SD and sample size.

Putting it another way, because every measurement is subject to some degree of error, every sample mean we calculate will be somewhat different. Most of the time, the sample means will cluster closely to the population mean, but every so often, we'll end up with a screwball result that differs from the truth just by chance. So if we drew a sample, did something to it, and measured the effect, we'd have a problem. If the mean differs from the population mean, is it because our intervention really had an effect, or is it because this is one of those rare times when we drew some oddballs? We can

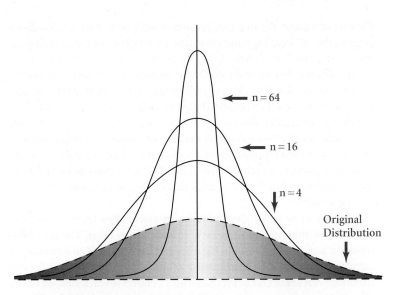

Figure 3-1 Original distribution and distribution of means related to sample size.

never be sure, but statistics tell a lot about how often we can expect the group to differ *by chance alone* (more on this later).

THE CENTRAL LIMIT THEORY

There's another key point in the notion of the SE of the mean, contained in those three little words "of the mean." Just about everything we do in statistical inference (at least up to Chapter 6) has to do with differences between means. We use the original data to estimate the mean of the sample and its SE and work forward from there.

It seems that most people who have taken a stats course forget this basic idea when they start to worry about when to use parametric statistics such as *t* tests. Although it is true that parametric statistics hang on the idea of a normal distribution, all we need is a normal distribution *of the means*, not of the original data.

Think about this one a little more. The basic idea of all of this is that the results of any one experiment are influenced by the operation of chance. If we did the experiment a zillion times and calculated the mean each time, these mean values would form some distribution centered on the true "population" mean with an SD equal to the original SD divided by the square root of the sample size. This would seem to imply that the *data* must be normally distributed if we're going to use this approach. Strangely, this is not so.

Time for a break. Let's talk football. All those giants (mere mortals inflated by plastic and foam padding) grunt out on the field in long lines at the start of a game. Because they're covered with more stuff than medieval knights, they all wear big numbers stitched on the back of their bulging jerseys so we can tell who's who. Typically, the numbers range from 1 to 99.

It turns out that we really don't like spectator sports, so if you gave us season tickets to the local NFL games, likely as not, we would sit there dreaming up some statistical diversion to keep ourselves amused. For example, let's test the hypothesis that the average number of each team is the same. (Boy, we must be bored!) We would sit on the 50-yard line, and as the lads ran onto the field, we would rapidly add their team numbers and then divide by the number of players on each side. We could do this for every game and gradually assemble a whole bunch of team means. Now, what would those numbers look like?

Well, we know the original numbers are essentially a rectangular distribution—any number from 1 to 99 is as likely as any other. The actual distribution generated is shown in Figure 3-2. It has a mean of 49.6. Would the calculated means also be distributed at random from 1 to 99 with a flat distribution? Not at all! Our bet is that, with 11 players on each side, we would almost never get a mean value less than 40 or more than 60 because, on the average, there would be as many numbers below 50 as above 50, so the mean of the 11 players would tend to be close to 50.

In Figure 3-3, we've actually plotted the distribution of means for 100 samples of size 11 drawn at random from a flat (rectangular) distribution ranging from 1 to 99. These data certainly look like a bell-shaped curve. The

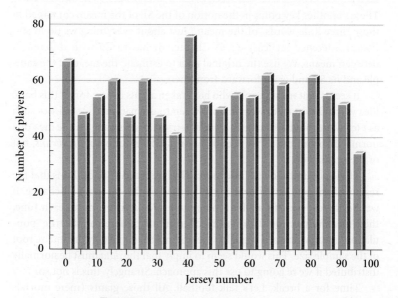

Figure 3-2 Distribution of original jersey numbers.

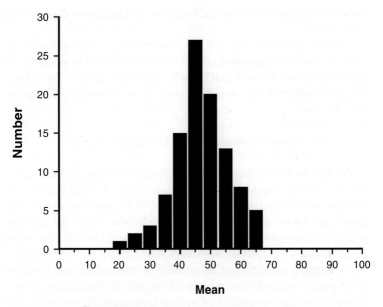

Figure 3-3 Distribution of means of sample size = 11.

calculated mean of this distribution is 49.62 (the same, naturally), and the SE is 8.86. If we had pretended that the original distribution was normal, not rectangular, the SD would have equaled 28. The SE would have been $28/\sqrt{11} = 8.45$, which is not far from 8.86.

Therein lies the magic of one of the most forgotten theorems in statistics: the **Central Limit Theorem**, which states that for sample sizes sufficiently large (and large means greater than 5 or 10), the means will be normally distributed *regardless of the shape of the original distribution*. So if we are making inferences on means, we can use parametric statistics to do the computations, whether or not the original data are normally distributed.

INFERENCES ABOUT MEAN VALUES BASED ON A SINGLE SAMPLE

Let's try to clarify this basic idea of statistics with a specific illustration. Consider an experiment that may have a direct bearing on how well you understand what's to come. We have written the book on the assumption that the average reader has an intelligence quotient (IQ) greater than 100. If we were wrong, then readers would not be able to decipher these ramblings, and our royalties wouldn't buy us a Big Mac. So we'd like some reassurance that we've targeted the book about right. How will we test this hypothesis?

To begin with, we'll do as all good researchers are supposed to do and rephrase it as a **null hypothesis**; that is to say, we'll start off by assuming that the readers are no different in IQ than the population at large. We will then do our darnedest to reject this hypothesis. So we phrase the null hypothesis as follows:

H_0: mean IQ of readers = mean IQ of general population

We have deliberately chosen an experiment involving IQ tests because they are carefully standardized on very large samples to have a normal distribution with a mean of 100 and an SD of 15. So, when we state the null hypothesis, we are assuming momentarily that the readers are a random sample of this population and have a true average IQ of 100. This sounds weird because that's what we don't want to be the case, but bear with us.

Continuing along this line of reasoning, we then assume that if we sample 25 readers repeatedly, give them an IQ test, and calculate their mean score, these calculated means would be distributed symmetrically around the population mean of 100. The question remains, "What is the expected random variation of these mean values?" Well, from the discussion in the previous section, the SE of these means is the SD of the original distribution divided by the square root of the sample size. In our case, this is $15/\sqrt{25} = 3.0$.

So, suppose we went ahead with the experiment involving 25 readers (we may have to give away a few complimentary copies to pull it off) and found their mean IQ to be 107.5. We want to determine the likelihood of obtaining a sample mean IQ of 107.5 or greater from a random sample of the population with a true mean of 100 (Figure 3-4). What we are seeking is the area in the tail to the right of 107.5. The way we approach it is to calculate the ratio of (107.5 − 100), or 7.5, to the SE of 3.0.

The ratio, 7.5/3.0 = 2.5, tells us how far we are out on the standard normal distribution; we then consult a table of values of the normal distribution and find out that the area in the tail is 0.006. Thus, the likelihood of obtaining a sample IQ of 107.5 or greater by chance, under the null hypothesis that the two population means are equal, is 0.006, or approximately 1 in 160. Because there is a low probability of obtaining a value this large or larger by chance, we *reject the null hypothesis* and conclude that the readers, with their average IQ of 107.5, are drawn from a different population (that is, they really do have an IQ greater than 100).

This approach of comparing a sample mean with a known population mean by calculating the ratio of the difference between means to the SE is known as the *z* **test**.

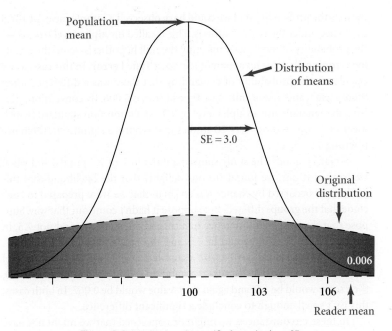

Population mean

Distribution of means

SE = 3.0

Original distribution

0.006

100   103   106

Reader mean

Figure 3-4 Distribution of mean IQ of sample size = 25.

TYPE I AND TYPE II ERRORS, ALPHA-LEVELS AND BETA-LEVELS, AND OTHER RULES OF STATISTICAL ETIQUETTE

The example we just worked through illustrates a couple of basic rules of the game of statistical inference. The starting point is almost always to assume that there is no difference between the groups; they are all samples drawn at random from the same statistical population. The next step is to determine the likelihood that the observed differences could be caused by chance variation alone. If this probability is sufficiently small (usually less than 1 in 20), then you "reject" the null hypothesis and conclude that there is some true difference between the groups. So, you are concluding that the independent variable (IV) had some effect on the dependent variable (DV) and that the samples therefore came from different populations, the "alternative hypothesis" (H_1). That is the meaning behind all those $p < 0.05$s and $p < 0.0001$s that appear in the literature. They are simply statements of the probability that the observed difference could have arisen by chance.

Going back to the "reader IQ" experiment, we concluded that the population IQ of readers was greater than 100. Suppose, to carry on the demonstration, that it was actually 110 and not 107.5, the sample estimate. The distribution of sample means of size 25 drawn from the two populations (readers and the general population) could then be pictured as in Figure 3-5. The small area from the general population curve to the right of the sample mean is the probability that we could have observed a sample mean of 107.5 by chance under the null hypothesis. This is called the **alpha level** (αlevel)—the probability of incorrectly rejecting the null hypothesis—and the resulting error is called, for no apparent reason, a **Type I error**. In this case, as we calculated, the probability of concluding that there was a difference when there wasn't, and of committing a Type I error, is 0.006. By convention, statisticians generally use an alpha level of 0.05 as a minimum standard (which means that one out of every 20 studies that reports a significant difference is wrong).

So far, so good. The study showed a difference of 7.5 points, and when we worked it out, we found (to our delight) that the likelihood that this could have occurred by chance was so small that we were prepared to conclude that the groups differed. But suppose it hadn't come out that way. Suppose that the observed difference had turned out to be 4.5 and not 7.5, in which case the z score would be 1.5 and the probability would be 0.067. Alternatively, if we had started with a sample size of 9, not 25, the alpha level would be more than 0.05 because the standard error would be $15 / \sqrt{9} = 5.0$, the z score would be 1.5, and again the p value would be 0.067. In both cases, this isn't small enough to conclude a significant difference.

In these circumstances, we might be concerned that we might not have had a big enough sample to detect a meaningful difference. How do we figure out whether we actually had a chance at detecting a meaningful difference? To work this one out, we have to first decide what is a meaningful difference, a task that has had monastic philosophers engaged in solemn

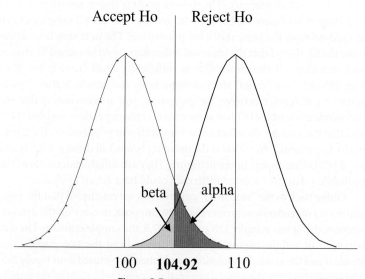

Accept Ho   Reject Ho

beta   alpha

100   **104.92**   110

Figure 3-5 Alpha and beta errors.

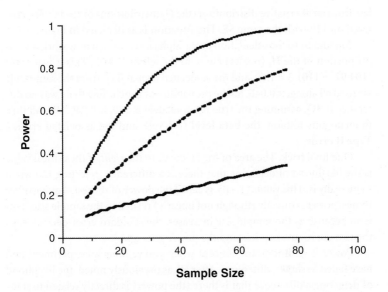

Figure 3-6 Relationship between power and difference between means, standard deviation, and sample size.

contemplation since medieval times. For obvious reasons, then, we won't get into that particular debate here. One quick rule of thumb in such quandaries is to say "10%." So let's suppose we wanted to detect a difference of 10 points (or 5, or 20, or 15—the choice is yours)…

The next step is to figure out exactly the circumstances under which we would either declare "significant difference" or "no difference." That is, if we look at the H_0 distribution in Figure 3-5, there is a critical value to the right of the mean, so that exactly 0.05 of the distribution is to the right of it and 0.95 is to the left of it. And if the observed mean falls to the right of it, then the alpha level is less than 0.05, and we party. If the mean is to the left of the critical value, we skulk off and drown our sorrows. (Note that whatever the conclusion, we get to have a drink.)

So where is this critical value? If we go back to the same table that gave us the z values (in some real stats book), we can work backwards from a p of 0.05 to discover that this equals a z value of 1.64. Since the SE is 3.0, the critical value is $1.64 \times 3 = 4.92$. So if the observed mean falls to the right of 4.92, it's "significant"; to the left, it's not.

If we now turn to the "meaningful difference" of 110, the question we want to ask as statisticians is, "What is the likelihood that we would have failed to detect a difference of 10 points?" or, more precisely, "What is the likelihood that we would have ended up with an observed mean of 4.92 or less from an alternative distribution (the H_1 distribution) of reader IQs, centered on 110 with the same SE. The situation is as depicted in Figure 3-5.

Analogous to the calculation of the alpha level, we can now work out the proportion of the H_1 (reader) curve to the left of 104.92. This is just a z of $(104.92 - 110)/3 = 1.69$, and the associated probability, from the same table we used all along, is 0.046. So the probability of concluding there was no difference in IQ, assuming the true IQ of readers is 110, is 0.046. We call this, in analogous fashion, the **beta level** (β-level), and the associated error, a **Type II error**.

One final trick. The area of the H_1 curve to the *right* of the critical value is the likelihood of declaring that there is a difference (rejecting H_0) when there really is. This value, $(1 - \beta)$, is called the **power** of the test. Among other things, power is directly (though not linearly) related to the sample size. This is so because as the sample size increases, the standard error decreases, so the two curves overlap less and the power goes up.

Power is an important concept when you've done an experiment and have failed to show a difference. After all, as previously noted, the likelihood of detecting a difference that is there (the power) is directly related to sample size. If a sample is too small, you can't show that anything is statistically significant, whereas if a sample is too big, everything is statistically significant. All this is shown in Figure 3-6. As our first stats prof used to say, "With a big sample, you're doomed to statistical significance."

However, if the difference is not significant, all those yea-sayers (who really want to show that the newest, latest, and most expensive drug really is better) will automatically scream, "Ya didn't have enough power, dummy!" Don't panic! As you can see from the preceding discussion, it is evident that power depends not only on sample size but also on the size of the difference you want to detect. And because the experiment did not reject the null hypothesis, you have no more idea of how much the "true" difference is than you did before you started. After all, if you knew that, there would be no reason to do the study. So, if you guess at a really big difference, you will find enough power.

Conversely, on one occasion, when we had reported a significant difference at the < 0.001 level with a sample size of approximately 15 per group, one intellectually challenged reviewer took us to task for conducting studies with such small samples, saying we didn't have enough power. Clearly, we did have enough power to detect a difference because we *did* detect it.

One final wrinkle to really test your mettle. Imagine that you have just completed an experiment (for the sake of argument, with two groups and measurements of IQ). You have just calculated the appropriate significance test, and it works out to a probability of 0.049999. Appropriately, you reject the null hypothesis and declare a significant difference. What is the likelihood that if you repeated the experiment exactly as before, you would come to the same conclusion and reject the null hypothesis? Most people say 95%.

In fact, this question is posed to our stats class every year, with $2.00 going to anyone who gets the answer. So far, it has cost us $4.00. The answer, believe it or not, is exactly 0.50; that is, if the experiment rejected H_0 at exactly the 0.05 level, the chance of replicating the experiment is 50%! To see why, look at Figure 3-7.

Well, not *exactly* 0.50. A very astute reader challenged us on this point just before this edition came out. He pointed out that we are assuming, in our logic, that H_1 is correct. But there is still a chance that H_0 is correct. The relative probabilities of each are measured by the height of the two curves: H_0 at $z = 1.96$ and H_1 at $z = 0$, which turn out to be about 0.05 and 0.40. So the actual probability of rejecting H_0 a second time is $[(0.40 \times 0.50) + (0.05 \times 0.05)] / (0.40 + 0.05) = 0.45$.

ONE-TAILED TESTS AND TWO-TAILED TESTS

Until now, we have only considered the possibility that readers were smarter than the general population. This conclusion would be accepted if the sample mean were sufficiently large that the probability in the right tail of the null hypothesis distribution was less than 5%. Because the hypothesis involves only one tail of the distribution, this is called a "one-tailed" test.

However, the occasion may arise (for example, in comparing two treatments) in which we do not want to declare the direction of the difference ahead of time but will be satisfied if a significant difference in either

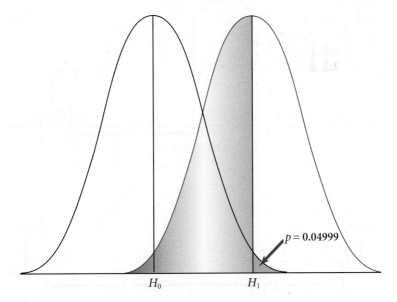

$p = 0.04999$

H_0 H_1

Figure 3-7 The probability of a second significant result after the first study is significant.

direction is obtained; so, if one treatment is better than or worse than the other by a sufficient amount, we will reject the null hypothesis. This amount must be determined by the probability in both tails of the distribution and therefore is called a "two-tailed" test.

What's the difference? In the two-tailed test, if we want to maintain an overall alpha level of 0.05, we can allow only half of this amount, or 0.025 in each tail. As a result, the difference between means must be larger in order to reject the null. For the z test, a difference of 1.64 SDs is significant at the 0.05 level for a one-tailed test, but a two-tailed test requires a difference of 1.96 SDs (Figure 3-8).

In real life, nearly all statistical analyses use two-tailed tests. Even when comparing a drug with a placebo, people act as if they would be equally pleased to find that the drug is significantly better or worse than the placebo. The explanation for this bizarre behavior lies not in the realm of logic but in science. If researchers did a trial of a drug and placebo by using a one-tailed test and if, for some reason, the drug bumped off more people than the placebo (don't laugh—it happens. Who can forget clofibrate?), they would be forced to conclude that these excess deaths were due to chance.

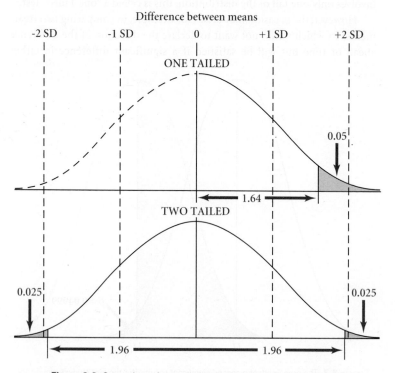

Figure 3-8 Comparison of one-tailed and two-tailed tests of significance.

CONFIDENCE INTERVALS

In the previous discussion, we put our data up against two hypotheses: (1) The mean population IQ of readers is 100, and (2) the mean IQ of readers is 110. Once the study is over, however, our best guess at the population IQ is not 100 or 110 but the value we determined from the study, 107.5. Nevertheless, there is some uncertainty in this estimate, which must be related to the SE of the mean, 3.0.

This relationship is clarified in Figure 3-9. Imagine first that the true population mean is 1.96 SEs below 107.5, or 101.6. In this instance, there is only a 2.5% probability that we could have obtained a sample IQ as high as 107.5 = 1.96 SEs. Similarly, if the true mean was 113.4, there is a 2.5% probability that we could obtain a sample IQ as low as 107.5. Turning the whole argument around, we might say that having obtained a sample IQ of 107.5, there is a 95% probability that the true population IQ lies between 101.6 and 113.4. This range is called a "95% confidence interval"; that is, we are 95% confident that the population mean lies in this interval. The 95% confidence interval is calculated as follows:

95% confidence interval = sample mean ± 1.96 × SE

If you regularly read the newspaper, you have actually encountered the 95% confidence interval in another guise. Every time Gallup, Angus Reed, or some other pollster proclaims that "Thirty-seven percent of Americans would vote for Lassie as the next president," they always add something like

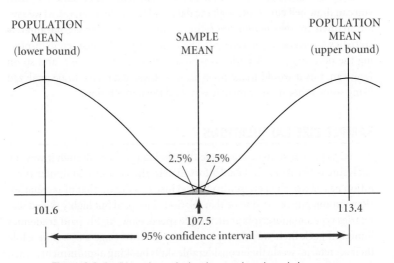

Figure 3-9 Confidence interval related to sample and population means.

"This poll is accurate to ± 3.2 points 95% of the time." That, you now know, is the 95% confidence interval. What, pray tell, did you think it was before you read this chapter?

There is a natural link between the confidence interval and hypothesis testing. Looking at Figure 3-9, if the lower limit of the confidence interval was exactly 100, then the left-hand curve is identical to the null hypothesis distribution. So, if the confidence interval includes the mean of the null hypothesis, then this is equivalent to not rejecting the null hypothesis.

PARAMETRIC AND NONPARAMETRIC STATISTICS

Now that we have the basic idea about statistical inference, and just before we leap in with both feet, a further bit of terminology. Statisticians often refer to two different kinds of statistical tests by using the obscure labels "parametric statistics" and (naturally enough) "nonparametric statistics." The former includes the stuff of Chapters 4 to 9—t tests, analysis of variance, regression analysis, analysis of covariance, and time series. The latter covers stuff like chi-square, logistic regression, and log-linear analysis, which are discussed in Chapters 10 to 12.

The basic difference is that, in parametric statistics, the DV is some measured quantity (a ratio or interval level variable), so it makes sense to calculate means and SDs. With nonparametric stats, the DV is usually either a count or ranking (such as of dead bodies, which happen often, or cures, which happen rarely) for which it makes no sense to calculate means (eg, "The average religion of Americans is 2.67").

Why the fancy names? Well, if you can calculate means and SDs, then you can draw bell curves through the data, and the normal curves, as we saw, are defined by two *parameters*—the mean and SD—hence, **parametric statistics**. Conversely, you can't put a bell curve through a histogram displaying the percentage of Americans who are Protestant, Catholic, and so on (you can, but it would make no sense). So these data have to be analyzed using some other nonparametric way, and the name follows.

SAMPLE SIZE CALCULATIONS

It used to be that statisticians made their living (pittance though it was) by analyzing other people's data. Unfortunately, the personal computer revolution has encroached on our livelihood just as it did on that of secretaries. (Revolution, nuts! It used to be that relatively low-paid but highly skilled secretaries typed manuscripts at incredible speed. Now, highly paid academics hunt and peck their way through manuscripts two fingers at a time while their secretaries waste their considerable skills booking appointments. Such is progress.) Anyway, we statisticians are an adaptive species, so we've found a new career—calculating sample sizes. Nowadays, no grant proposal gets to square one without a sample size calculation. And if by some fluke you get the study funded without one, the ethics committee will want to see one before they let you near the first patient, anyway. So take a number, and line up at the door.

To be honest, sample size calculations are the most tedious part of the job. As we will see, they are based on nothing but a hope and a prayer because they require some heroic assumptions about the likely differences you will encounter at the end of the study. In fact, the only time you are really in a good position to do a defensible sample size calculation is after the study is over because only then will you have decent estimates of the required parameters.

Failing that, it's possible to get about any size of sample you could ever want. As we will show you, every sample size calculation involves separate estimates of four different quantities in order to arrive at the fifth, the sample size. The real talent that statisticians bring to the situation is the ability to fiddle all those numbers through several iterations so that the calculated sample size precisely equals the number of patients you wanted to use in the first place. We always give people what they want when it comes to sample size; that's why we're paid so well now.

To save you all those consultation bucks, we're about to reveal our secrets (kind of like the magician showing how the woman gets sawed in half). We start with the two normal curves of Figure 3-5. A moment's reflection reveals that the shape of those curves is determined by the following four quantities:

1. The distance between the two mean values, which we'll call *d*.
2. The width of the two curves (assumed to be the same). This equals the SD, *s*, divided by the square root of the sample size, *n*.
3. The distance from the left-hand curve (the null hypothesis) to the critical value (in Figure 3-5, it's 4.92). This is in turn related to the choice of the alpha level (0.05, 0.10, or whatever).
4. The distance from the right-hand curve (the alternate hypothesis) to the critical value (in Figure 3-5, it's 5.08), and this is related to the choice of the beta level.

If we know any three of the four numbers, we can determine the fourth analytically. So if we fix the difference between the two means, the SD, the sample size, and the alpha level, then we can determine the beta level. That's what we did in the previous section, but it also works the other way. If we fix the alpha level and beta level, the difference between the two means, and the SD, then this determines the sample size.

That's how sample size calculations proceed. We take guesses (occasionally educated, more commonly wild) at the difference between means and the SD, fix the alpha and beta levels at some arbitrary figures, and then crank out the sample size. The dialogue between the statistician and a client may go something like this:

Statistician: So, Dr. Doolittle, how big a treatment effect do you think you'll get?

Dr. Doolittle: I dunno, stupid. That's why I'm doing the study.

S: Well, how do 10 points sound?

D: Sure, why not?

S: And what is the standard deviation of your patients?

D: Excuse me. I'm an internist, not a shrink. None of my patients are deviant.

S: Oh well, let's say 15 points. What alpha level would you like?

D: Beats me.

S: 0.05 as always. Now please tell me about your beta?

D: I bought a VHS machine years ago.

S: Well, we'll say point 2. (Furiously punches calculator.) You need a sample size of 36.

D: Oh, that's much too big! I only see five of those a year.

S: Well, let's see. We could make the difference bigger. Or the standard deviation smaller. Or the alpha level higher. Or the beta level higher. Where do you want to start fudging?

The actual formula is a bit hairy, but we can guess what it might look like from the picture. The bigger the difference, the smaller the required sample size, so the difference between groups must be in the denominator. The bigger the SD, the larger the required sample size, so the SD must be in the numerator. You really don't have much to say about the alpha level; unless you are really desperate, that has to be 0.05. Finally, if you are willing to forego the opportunity to mess around with the beta level and accept a standard beta level of 0.2 (a power of 80%), which is as low as you should dare go anyway, then the whole mess reduces to the following easy formula[1]:

$$n = 16 \frac{s^2}{d^2}$$

So, taking the above example, with a difference (*d*) of 10, an SD (*s*) of 15, and alpha and beta as required, the sample size is as follows:

$$n = 16 \frac{s^2}{d^2} = 16 \times \left(\frac{15}{10}\right)^2 = 36$$

Amazing how much they will pay us to do this little trick.

Regrettably, the world is a bit more complicated than that because this formula only works when you have two groups and a continuous DV, so we have to devise some alternatives for other more complicated cases. To do so, we will be using terms such as analysis of variance (ANOVA) and regression, which you won't encounter until later, so you may have to take some of this on faith.

---

[1]Lehr R. Sixteen S-squared over D-squared: a relation for crude sample size estimates. *Stat Med* 1992;11:1099–102.

The following are strategies for some other situations:

1. Difference between proportions (see Chapter 9). Often, people like to do studies where they count bodies at the end and see whether the latest (and most expensive) drug can save lives. They end up comparing the proportion of people in the drug group (Pd) with the proportion in the placebo group (Pp). The sample size equation uses the difference between the two ($Pp - Pd$) in the denominator. However, the SD is calculated directly from the average of the proportions—($Pp + Pd$)/2, which we will call p, using some arcane theory of numbers—resulting in the following modified formula:

$$n = \frac{16\,[p(1-p)]}{(Pp - Pd)^2}$$

2. Difference among many means (see Chapter 5). Although there are exact methods to calculate sample sizes when you have many means and are using ANOVA methods, these involve additional assumptions about the way the means are distributed and are even less defensible (if that's possible). What we do is pick the one comparison between the two means that we care the most about, and then use the original formula.

3. Relation between two continuous variables (see Chapter 6). Calculating sample size for a regression coefficient involves knowledge of both the coefficient and its SE, at which no mortal can hazard a guess. A better way is to do the calculation on the correlation coefficient, r. As it turns out, the SD of a correlation coefficient is approximately equal to $1/\sqrt{(n-2)}$, so to test whether this differs from zero (the usual situation), we can again manipulate the original formula, and it becomes strangely different:

$$n = 4 + \frac{8}{r}$$

4. Relation among many variables (see Chapters 6, 7, 8, and 13 to 19). At this point, we throw up our hands and invoke an old rule of thumb—the sample size should be 5 to 10 times the number of variables.

    Looks like we just did ourselves out of a job. One final caveat, though: sample size calculations should be used to tell you the order of magnitude you need—whether you need 10, 100, or 1,000 people, not whether you need 22 or 26.

STATISTICAL VERSUS CLINICAL SIGNIFICANCE

In a preceding section, we established the basic link between the magnitude of an observed difference and the calculated probability that such a difference could have arisen by chance alone. The game plan is to determine this probability, and if it is sufficiently small, to conclude that the difference was unlikely to have occurred by chance alone. We then end up saying something like, "Readers of the book are *significantly* smarter than the general population."

And that is the meaning behind **statistical significance**; that is, the probability of the observed difference arising by chance was sufficiently small, and therefore, we can conclude that the IV had some effect. It's really too bad that someone in the history of statistics decided to call this phenomenon "statistical significance" as opposed to, say, "a statistically nonzero effect" or "a statistically present effect" because the term is, somehow, so significant. The basic notion has been perverted to the extent that $p < 0.05$ has become the holy grail of clinical and behavioral research, and that $p < 0.0001$ is cause to close the lab down for the afternoon and declare a holiday.

Let's take a closer look at what determines that magical p level. Three variables enter into the determination of a z score (and as we shall see, nearly every other statistical test): (1) the observed difference between means, (2) the SD of the distribution, and (3) the sample size. A change in any one of these three values can change the calculated statistical significance. As an example, we can examine the results of the reader IQ experiment for sample sizes of 4 to 10,000. How would this variation in sample size affect the size of difference necessary to achieve $p < 0.05$ (that is, statistical significance)? Table 3-1 displays the results.

So a difference of 10 IQ points with a sample size of 4 is just as significant, statistically, as a difference of 0.2 IQ points for a sample size of 10,000. We don't know about you, but we would probably pay $100.00 for a correspondence course that raised IQ by 10 points (from 140 to 150, of course), but we wouldn't part with a dime for a course that was just as statistically significant but raised IQ by only two-tenths of a point.

Table 3-1
Relationship of Sample Size and Mean Values to Achieve Statistical Significance

Sample Size	Reader Mean	Population	p
4	110.0	100.0	0.05
25	104.0	100.0	0.05
64	102.5	100.0	0.05
400	101.0	100.0	0.05
2,500	100.4	100.0	0.05
10,000	100.2	100.0	0.05

Sample size has a similar impact on the beta level. If the true IQ of readers was 119, a sample of 4 would have a beta level of 0.37; that is, only a 63% chance of detecting it. The beta level for a sample of 100 is 0.05 and for a sample of 10,000 is less than 0.0001. So, if the sample is too small, you risk the possibility of not detecting the presence of real effects.

The bottom line is this: the level of statistical significance—0.05, 0.001, or whatever—indicates the likelihood that the study could have come to a false conclusion. By itself, it tells you *absolutely nothing* about the actual magnitude of the differences between groups.

Up to now, we haven't talked about clinical significance. Basically, this reduces to a judgment by someone of how much of a difference might be viewed as clinically important. The topic consumes zillions of journal pages in the Health-Related Quality of Life literature, basically because no one can agree anyway. However, Jacob Cohen, a statistician and pragmatist, framed differences in terms of a simple concept called the **effect size** (mean difference / standard deviation of the sample) and said, based on reviewing some literature, that a small effect size was about 0.2, a medium one was about 0.5, and a large one was about 0.8. That seems to be as good as any other approach.

C.R.A.P. DETECTORS

Example 3-1

The Lipids Research Clinics (LRC) Trial screened 300,000 men to find 3,000 with cholesterol levels in the top 1%, no heart disease, and high compliance with the treatment regimen. They randomized the sample to active drug and placebo regimens and, after 10 years, found 38 cardiac deaths in the controls and 30 in the drug group ($p < 0.05$). A margarine company then proclaimed that everybody should switch from butter to margarine to prevent heart disease.

Question. Given your new knowledge, would you switch?

Answer. This is a real perversion of the large sample. First, the effect of the drug is statistically significant but clinically trivial. Second, the results may apply to folks who are similar to those studied, but they don't apply to (1) women, (2) individuals with lower cholesterol levels, and (3) margarine users. This example, alas, actually occurred.

C.R.A.P. Detector III-1

Beware the large sample. Effects can be statistically significant and clinically inconsequential.

C.R.A.P. Detector III-2

Beware the sweeping generalization. The results of any study apply only to populations similar to the study sample.

Example 3-2

A rheumatologist studied the effect of copper bracelets on 10 patients with arthritis. He measured 26 variables and found a significant lowering of blood levels but no effect on pain or function. He concluded that copper can affect blood levels of rheumatoid factor but nothing else.

Question. Do you believe him?

Answer. Here's a small-sample beauty. First, with 10 patients, it's unlikely to have enough power to show anything. So all the rheumatologist can safely say about the 25 other variables is that he was unable to demonstrate a difference and not that there wasn't one. Actually, you can never prove the null hypothesis. Second, with 26 tests, one may be significant by change alone and so mean nothing.

C.R.A.P. Detector III-3

Beware the small sample. It's hard to find significant differences, and no difference means nothing.

C.R.A.P. Detector III-4

Multiple comparisons are a statistical no-no! There are special ways to handle these kinds of data.

4

Comparison of Means of Two Samples: The *t* Test

The *t* test is used for measured variables in comparing two means. The *unpaired t test* compares the means of two independent samples. The *paired t test* compares two paired observations on the same individual or on matched individuals.

In our discussion of the *z* test, we used as a dependent variable (DV) an intelligence quotient (IQ) test, which has a known mean and standard deviation (SD), in order to compare our sample of interest —namely, readers of this magnificent opus—to the general population. We did not have to scrape up a control group of nonreaders for comparison because we knew in advance the true mean and SD of any control group we might draw from the general population.

This fortunate circumstance rarely occurs in the real world. As a result, many studies involve a comparison of two groups, treatment versus control, or treatment A versus treatment B. The statistical analysis of two samples is a bit more complicated than the previous comparison between a sample and a population. Previously, we used the population SD to estimate the random error we could expect in our calculated sample mean. In a two-sample comparison, this SD is not known and must be estimated from the two samples.

Let's consider a typical randomized trial of an antihypertensive drug. We locate 50 patients suffering from hypertension, randomize them into two groups, institute a course of drug or placebo, and measure the diastolic blood pressure. We then calculate a mean and SD for each group. Suppose the results are as shown in Table 4-1.

The statistical question is "What is the probability that the difference of 4 mm Hg between treatment and control groups could have arisen by chance?" If this probability is small enough, then we will assume that the

Table 4-1
Typical Randomized Trial

	Treatment Group	Control Group
Sample size	25	25
Mean	98 mm Hg	102 mm Hg
Standard deviation	6 mm Hg	8 mm Hg

difference is not due to chance and that there is significant effect of the drug on blood pressure.

To approach this question, we start off with a null hypothesis that the population values of the two groups are not different. Then we try to show they are different. If we were to proceed as before, we would calculate the ratio of the difference between the two means, 4 mm Hg, to some estimate of the error of this difference. In Chapter 3, we determined the standard error (SE) as the population SD divided by the square root of the sample size; but this time, the population SD is unknown. We do, however, have two estimates of this population value, namely, the sample SDs calculated from the treatment and control groups. One approach to getting a best estimate of the population SD would be to average the two values. For reasons known only to statisticians, a better approach is to add the squares of the SDs to give $6^2 + 8^2 = 36 + 64 = 100$. The next step is to divide this variance by the sample size and take the square root of the result to obtain the SE:

$$SE = \sqrt{(100/25)} = 2.0$$

As usual, then, to determine the significance of this difference, you take the ratio of the calculated difference to its SE.

$$t = \frac{\text{difference between means}}{\text{SE of difference}} = 4.0/2.0 = 2.0$$

The probability we are looking for is the area to the right of 4 mm Hg on the curve (that is, 2.0×2 mm Hg), which is close to 0.025 (one-tailed) (Figure 4-1).

The above formula works fine if the two samples are of equal size. However, if there are unequal samples, and you look in a real statistics book, you will find a complicated formula sprinkled liberally with n's and $n-1$'s. The basis for the formula, and the reason for its complexity, is twofold: (1) if one sample is bigger than the other, the estimated variance from it is more accurate, so it should weigh more in the calculation of the SE; and (2) because the SE involves a division by n, the formula has to account for the fact that there are now two n's kicking around. Don't worry about it; computers know the formula.

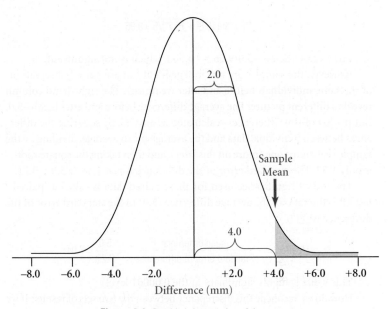

Figure 4-1 Graphic interpretation of the *t* test.

This test statistic is called the **Student's *t* test**. It was developed by the statistician William Gossett, who was employed as a quality control supervisor at the Guinness Brewery in Dublin and who wrote under the pseudonym of Student, presumably because no one who knew his occupation would take him seriously. It turns out that this curve is not a normal curve when you get to small samples, so you have to look it up in a different appendix, under the "*t*" distribution.

THE PAIRED *t* TEST

Before you knew anything about research design, you might have approached the hypertension trial somewhat differently. The most obvious way to do the experiment is to measure the diastolic pressure in a group of patients, give them the drug, and then measure blood pressure again a month or two later. Suppose we measured five patients, whose raw data are presented in Table 4-2.

For a moment, let's ignore the fact that these are "before" and "after" measurements and assume they are data from two independent samples, with "before" representing the control group and "after" representing the treatment group. If we were to proceed with a *t* test as described in the previous section, the difference between means is −5.0. The standard error of this difference is as follows:

$$SE = \sqrt{(15.8^2 + 15.7^2)/5} = 9.96$$

The t value then is $-5.0/9.96 = -0.502$, which is not significant.

However, the samples are not independent but are paired observations of the same individuals before and after treatment. The right-hand column reveals a different picture. The average difference before and after is still -5.0. But the SD of this difference—calculated as any SD, by squaring the differences between individual data and the average mean average, dividing by the sample size minus one (more on this later), and then taking the square root—is only 1.58. The standard error of the difference is just $1.58/\sqrt{5.0} = 0.71$.

The test of significance used for these paired data is called a "paired t test." It is the ratio of the average difference (5.0) to the standard error of the difference (0.71).

$$t\,(\text{paired}) = \frac{\text{mean difference}}{\text{Standard error of differences}} = \frac{5.0}{0.71} = 7.04$$

This value is highly significant at the 0.00001 level.

How do we reconcile this discrepancy between the two sets of results? If we back up from all the mathematic gimcrackery of the last page or so and go back to the table of raw data, what the before-after observations succeed in doing is almost completely removing the effect of individual differences between subjects, resulting in an enormous increase in the precision of measurement.

It's easy to visualize any number of situations in which individual patients could be assessed both before and after treatment. If we were looking at the effectiveness of a diet for treatment of obesity, it would be natural to weigh people before they started the diet and to subtract this weight from their weight at the end. Similarly, if you want to try out an educational program to teach statistics to a heterogeneous group of health professionals and assess its effectiveness with a multiple-choice posttest, it would be a good idea to assess prior knowledge with a comparable pretest.

Table 4-2
Effect of Antihypertensive Agent on Diastolic Blood Pressure

Patient	Before Treatment	After Treatment	Difference
1	120.0	117.0	−3
2	100.0	96.0	−4
3	110.0	105.0	−5
4	90.0	84.0	−6
5	130.0	123.0	−7
Mean	110.0	105.0	−5.0
SD	15.0	15.7	1.58

Surprisingly, this design can also lead to a loss of power under some circumstances. Reflect for a minute on the things contributing to the denominator of the *t* test. As we indicated earlier, some of this noise comes from stable individual differences; the rest comes from variability within subjects, either error of measurement or natural variation. When you do a paired *t* test, you remove the former, but you double the contribution of the latter, once from the pretest and once from the posttest. So if the within-subject variation is larger than the between-subject variation, then the paired *t* test loses power.

It's worth a reminder that this experimental approach, although potentially more precise than a treatment-control design, cannot ascribe the observed difference, statistically significant or not, solely to the experimental treatment. The weight watchers may have concurrently run out of food or developed an allergy to pizza, and the health professionals, in their enthusiasm, may have gone out and bought a copy of this book.

THE TWO-GROUP PRETEST-POSTTEST DESIGN

Is there any way out of this dilemma? Can you have your cake and eat it too? Of course. All you have to do is allocate people to an experimental group and a control group, as you would with an ordinary randomized experiment, then do both a pretest and a posttest on them. That way, you can unambiguously claim that the observed differences are due to the intervention, while enjoying the potential gain in power from the pretest-posttest design.

The analysis is a combination of the paired and unpaired *t* tests. You take the differences between pretest and posttest in the two groups, just as if you were going to do a paired *t* test. Then you do an *unpaired t* test on the two sets of difference scores. That's all there is to it. By the way, what you *don't* do is a paired *t* test on the experimental groups and another one on the control group, and then if the first is significant and the second not, claim that you've proved your point. See Example 4-2.

One final point of particular relevance to the educators in our midst: in doing educational studies, people really like to do pretests and posttests, but they forget a serious design implication of the strategy. The pretest, to the extent that it reflects the content of the educational manipulation, tells everybody, in both the experimental and control group, what the course is all about (and if it doesn't reflect the course content, why do it?). It may result in folks in the experimental group focusing their learning on only exam-type content. It may also give the control group an idea of what they should study to kick the butts of the lucky people in the experimental group (the "John Henry" effect). Either way, the results are potentially biased in an unpredictable manner.

C.R.A.P. Detectors

Example 4-1

Another true horror story. Several years ago, a popular treatment for angina was to surgically ligate the internal mammary artery. Patients rated the degree of pain before and after surgery. A *t* test showed significant reduction in pain as a result of surgery. The conclusion drawn was that the therapy was effective.

Question. Are you a believer?

Answer. The small point is that the design demands a paired *t* test. When the test is not specified, it's usually unpaired, which is wrong. The big point, as was shown later by randomized trials in which the artery wasn't ligated in half of the patients, was that the result was due to placebo effect. The moral is that you always need a control group to prove causation.

C.R.A.P. Detector IV-1

To conclude that a difference between two groups or a difference within a group is due to some variable requires that the two samples differ only in the independent variable and in none other.

Example 4-2

Bennett and colleagues[1] used a randomized trial to improve students' knowledge of critical appraisal in two areas: diagnosis and therapeutics. They administered a pretest and a posttest in each area to the treatment group (which received training in critical appraisal) and to the control group (which did not). For the treatment group, the paired *t* test was highly significant ($p < 0.001$) for diagnosis and significant ($p < 0.01$) for therapy. For the control group, neither *t* test was significant. The investigators concluded that critical appraisal teaching works.

Question. Would you have analyzed the study this way?

Answer. Approaching the analysis this way essentially ignores the control group. The investigators should have done an *unpaired t* test on the difference scores, contrasting the treatment with the control group. In fact, the investigators reported both analyses.

C.R.A.P. Detector IV-2

First, any conclusion drawn from multiple tests causes a loss of control of the alpha level and is extremely difficult to interpret. Second, doing separate paired *t* tests on the treatment and control groups is statistically illogical.

---

[1]Bennett KJ et al. A controlled trial of teaching critical appraisal of the clinical literature to medical students. JAMA 1987;257:2451–4.

5

Comparison among Many Means: Analysis of Variance

Analysis of variance (ANOVA) allows comparison among more than two sample means. *One-way ANOVA* deals with a single categorical independent variable (or factor). *Factorial ANOVA* deals with multiple factors in many different configurations.

N*o doubt,* on the occasions when you sat in front of your television set for an evening, it must have occurred to you to ask whether there really was any difference among the products advertised on the commercials. Is Cottonbelle bathroom tissue really softer? Do floors shine better with new clear Smear? Does Driptame really stop postnasal drip? If you set out to do the experiment, one problem might be to pick two products to compare because in the case of bathroom tissue, dirty floors, and runny noses, there are many brand names from which to choose. The real question is not so much "Is Brand A better than Brand B?" but rather "Is there any measurable difference at all among the brands?" So instead of a single comparison between two groups, what we are after is some overall comparison among possibly many groups.

Let's be a bit more specific. Suppose, as a family physician, you are interested in determining whether there is a significant difference in pain-relieving characteristics among the many acetylsalicylic acid-based over-the-counter medications. A visit to the local drugstore convinces you to include six different medications in your study: five brand-name drugs and one generic drug. A first comparison that you might wish to make would be between the brand-name drugs and the generic drug (ie, five possible comparisons). But you also might wish to compare Brand A with Brand B, A with C, A with D, and so forth. If you work it out, there are 15 possible comparisons. If there were eight drugs, there would be 28 comparisons; 10 drugs, 45 comparisons; and so on. The rub is that 1 out of 20 comparisons will be significant by chance alone, at the 0.05 level, so pretty soon you can no longer tell the real differences from the chance differences. (Actually, with 15 comparisons, the likelihood that at least one comparison will be significant is already approximately 54%, thanks to the arcane laws of probability). The use of multiple t tests to do two-way comparisons is inappropriate because the process leads to a loss of any interpretable level of significance. What we need is a statistical method that permits us to make a statement about overall differences among drugs, following which we could seek out where the differences lie. Our null hypothesis (H_0) and alternative hypothesis (H_1) take the following forms:

H_0: All the means are equal.
H_1: Not all the means are equal.

We would proceed to assemble some patients, randomly allocate them to the six treatment groups, administer the various acetylsalicylic acid (ASA) preparations (each delivered in a plain brown wrapper), and then ask the patients to rate pain on a subjective scale from 0 = no pain to 15 = excruciating pain. The results of the experiment are shown in Table 5-1.

Five patients are assigned to each of the six groups. Each patient makes some pain rating (eg, 5.0 is the rating of patient 1 in the drug A group). The mean score in each group is obtained by averaging these ratings (eg, 7.0 is the mean rating in group A). Finally, we can obtain an overall mean, 8.0, from averaging all 30 ratings.

Now, if we want to know whether drug A stood out from the crowd, the first step is to find the difference between the mean pain score of drug A and the overall mean. Similarly, any difference between one drug and the rest can be detected by examining the difference between its group mean and the grand mean.

Table 5-1
Pain Ratings for Patients in Six Acetylsalicylic Acid Groups

Patient	A	B	Drug C	D	E	F
1	5.0	6.0	7.0	10.0	5.0	9.0
2	6.0	8.0	8.0	11.0	8.0	8.0
3	7.0	7.0	9.0	13.0	6.0	7.0
4	8.0	9.0	11.0	12.0	4.0	5.0
5	9.0	10.0	10.0	9.0	7.0	6.0
Mean	7.0	8.0	9.0	11.0	6.0	7.0
Overall mean = 8.0						

So to find the overall effect of the drugs, we take the differences between group means and the overall mean, square them (just as in the standard deviation) to get rid of the negative signs, and add them. The sum looks like the following:

$$(7 - 8)^2 + (8 - 8)^2 + (9 - 8)^2 + (11 - 8)^2 + (6 - 8)^2 + (7 - 8)^2 = 16.0$$

The sum is then multiplied by the number of subjects per group, 5, to obtain the **Sum of Squares (between groups)**:

Sum of Squares (between) = sum of (group mean − grand mean)^2 × N

In this case, it equals $16.0 \times 5 = 80$.

The next question is how to get an estimate of the variability within the groups. This is done by calculating the sum of the squared differences between individual values and the mean value within each group because this captures individual variability between subjects. Because this is based on variation within groups, it is called the **Sum of Squares (within groups)**:

Sum of Squares (within) = sum of (individual value − group mean)^2

$$= (5 - 7)^2 + (6 - 7)^2 + (7 - 7) + (8 - 7)^2 + (9 - 7)^2 + \ldots + (6 - 7)^2$$

There are 30 terms in this sum. The larger the Sum of Squares (between) relative to the Sum of Squares (within), the larger the difference between groups compared to the variation of individual values. However, the Sum of Squares (between groups) contains as many terms as there are groups, and the Sum of Squares (within groups) contains as many terms as there are individual data in all the groups. So the more groups, the larger the Sum of Squares (between), and the more data, the larger the Sum of Squares (within). Since what we're really trying to do is get the *average* variation between groups and compare it to the *average* variation within groups, it makes sense to divide the Sum of Squares (between) by the number of groups and divide the Sum of Squares (within) by the number of data.

Actually, at this point, a little more sleight of hand emerges. Statisticians start with the number of terms in the sum, then subtract the number of mean values that were calculated along the way. The result is called the **degrees of freedom**, for reasons that reside, believe it or not, in the theory of thermodynamics. Then, dividing the Sum of Squares by the degrees of freedom results in a new quantity called the **Mean Square**. Finally, the ratio of the two mean squares is a measure of the relative variation between groups of variation within groups and is called an *F* **ratio**.

F = mean square (between)/mean square (within)

The F test is something like a t test; that is, the bigger it is, the smaller the probability that the difference could occur by chance. And as with a t test, you have to look up the value of probability corresponding to the particular value in the back of a book (if the computer hasn't provided it for you). It has one important difference: the value depends on both the number of degrees of freedom (df) in the numerator and the denominator, so that the table lists both the numerator and denominator df. And it has one major similarity: if you do an analysis of variance (ANOVA) with only two groups, where you would expect the ANOVA to arrive at the same conclusion as the equivalent t test, it does. In fact, the value of the F test is the square of the equivalent t test.

This analysis is usually presented in an analysis of variance table, which looks something like Table 5-2.

The first column of Table 5-2 lists the Sums of Squares over which we agonized. The second column indicates the degrees of freedom, roughly equal to the number of terms in the Sum of Squares. The third column, the Mean Square, derives from dividing the Sum of Squares by degrees of freedom. Finally, the F test is the ratio of the two Mean Squares and can be looked up in yet another table at the back of the book. Because the method involves the analysis of only a single factor (eg, drug brand), it is called a **one-way ANOVA**.

These relationships may be presented graphically (Figure 5-1). Individual data from each group are shown to be normally distributed around each group mean, and all groups are projected downward onto an overall distribution centered on the grand mean of 8.0. Now the mean square (between) is related to the average difference between individual group means and the grand mean, and the greater the differences between groups, the larger this quantity. The mean square (within) comes from the difference between individual data and their group mean and so estimates the variance of the individual distributions. Finally, the F ratio is the ratio of these two quantities, so the larger the difference between groups, in comparison to their individual variance, the larger the F ratio and the more significant (statistically speaking) the result.

Let's go back to the initial question we posed. We wondered if there were any difference at all between various pain relievers. Having used ANOVA to

Table 5-2
Analysis of Variance

Source	Sum of Squares	Degrees of Freedom	Mean Square	F
Between groups	80.0	5	16.0	6.4
Within groups	60.0	24	2.5	—
Total	140.0	29	—	—

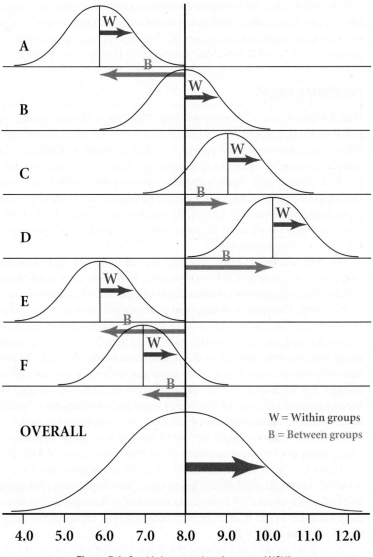

Figure 5-1 Graphic interpretation of one-way ANOVA.

satisfy ourselves that there is a significant difference somewhere in all that propaganda, the next likely question is "where?" Note that if the ANOVA does not turn up any overall differences, the rule is STOP! DO NOT PASS GO, DO NOT COLLECT $200, AND DO NOT DO ANY MORE NUMBER

CRUNCHING! But supposing the F value was significant, there are a number of procedures, called "post hoc comparisons," that can be used to find out where the significant differences lie. The use of a t test, even with a significant ANOVA, is still forbidden ground when there are many groups.

FACTORIAL ANOVA

If all ANOVA had to offer was a small edge over t tests in looking after significance levels, it wouldn't be worth all the effort involved in calculating it. But by an extension of the approach, called **factorial ANOVA**, we can include any number of factors in a single experiment and look at the independent effect of each factor without committing the cardinal sin of distorting the overall probability of a chance difference. As a bonus, by examining interactions between factors, we can also see whether, for example, some treatments work better on some types of subjects or have synergistic effects with other treatments.

To illustrate, let's examine that mainstay of midwinter television, the cough and cold remedy. Colds seem to come in two varieties, runny noses and hacking coughs. Some remedies like to take a broad-spectrum approach; at last count, Driptame was supposed to knock out 26 symptoms. Other brands try for "specificity"; Try-a-mine-ic eats up about 6 feet of drugstore shelf space with all the permutations to make you dry up or drip more, cough less or cough loose. All in all, an ideal situation for factorial ANOVA. The original question remains "Is there any difference overall among brands?" But some other testable questions come to mind, for example, "Do broad-spectrum remedies work better or worse than specific ones?" "Which kind of cold is more uncomfortable?" and "Do remedies work better or worse on runny noses or hacking cough?" Believe it or not, it's possible to have a swing at all of these questions at one time, using factorial ANOVA.

Here's how. Start out with, say, 100 folks with runny noses and 100 others with bad coughs. Half of each group uses a broad-spectrum (BS) agent, and half uses a specific (SP) remedy. In turn, half of these groups get Brand A, and half get Brand B, or 25 in each subgroup. The experimental design would look like Table 5-3.

Now if we get everyone to score the degree of relief on a 15-point scale, the mean of runny noses (RNs) is shown as 8.0 on the right, and the mean of hacking coughs (HCs) is 6.5. Similarly, the mean for Brand A is at the bottom, 6.0, as are the other brand means. Means for BS and SP drugs are shown on the last line and are the averages of the two brands in each group. Finally, we have indicated all the individual subgroup means. Sums of Squares for each factor can be developed as before by taking differences between individual group means and the grand mean, squaring, and summing. This is then mul-

Table 5-3
Experimental Design for Cold Remedy Study

| | Broad-Spectrum (BS) | | Specific (SP) | | |
	A	B	C	D	Mean
Runny noses (RNs)	7.5	8.5	9.0	7.0	8.0
Hacking coughs (HCs)	4.5	5.5	5.0	11.0	6.5
Mean (brands)	6.0	7.0	7.0	9.0	7.25
Mean (BS/SP)		6.5		8.0	

tiplied by a constant related to the number of levels of each factor in the design. For example, the Sum of Squares for BS versus SP drugs is as follows:

$$\text{Sum of Squares (BS/SP)} = [(6.5 - 7.25)^2 + (8.0 - 7.25)^2] \times 100 = 112.5$$

Mean squares can then be developed by dividing by the degrees of freedom—in this case, 1—as we did before. But there is still more gold in them thar hills, called **interaction terms**. As discussed, one would hope that relievers that are specific for drippy noses work better in the RN group and that those specific to coughs would be more helpful to HC members. That's a hypothesis about how the two factors go together or interact.

In Figure 5-2, we have displayed, on the left, the four cell means for the BS remedies. The center picture contains the cell means for the SP cures. Finally, the right graph looks at BS remedies against SP remedies by averaging across brands and plotting.

In the left picture, we see that overall, the BS drugs are more effective for RNs than HCs (8.0 vs 5.0) and that Brand B has an edge of 1 unit on Brand A. But there is no evidence of interaction, because the lines are parallel. In the jargon, this overall difference is called a **main effect** (in this case, a main effect of Brand A and a main effect of RN vs HC). By contrast, in the middle picture, Brand C, which was specific for RNs, works much better for RNs, and Brand D works better for HCs. Overall, Brand D is only a bit better than C. So this picture shows a strong interaction but little in the way of main effects. Finally, the right picture has a bit of both because SP and BS drugs are equally

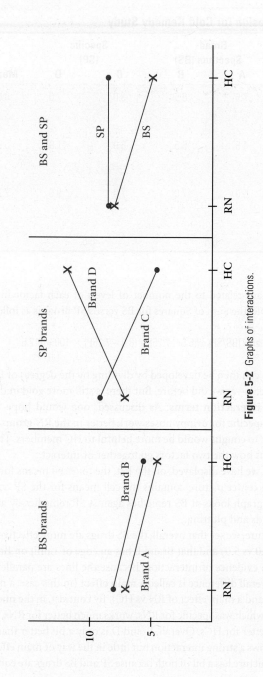

Figure 5-2 Graphs of interactions.

effective for RNs, but SP drugs work better for HCs. The important point is that useful information is often contained in the interaction terms—in this case, information about the very strong effect of SP drugs if they are used as intended, which would be lost in examining the overall effect of each factor.

The calculations become a bit hairy, but the general principle remains the same. The numerators for each effect are based on squared differences among mean values. The denominators, or error terms, are derived from squared differences between individual values and the appropriate mean. The end result is an expanded ANOVA table with one line for each main effect and interaction and an F ratio for each effect that indicates whether or not it was significant. Table 5-4 is an example of an ANOVA table from the present study.

The F ratio is like all our other tests in that the larger it is, the more statistically significant is the result. However, the associated probabilities are dependent on the number of terms in both numerator and denominator.

REPEATED MEASURES ANOVA

Just as we found that the paired t test, in which each subject was measured before and after some intervention, has some real advantages in statistical power (when the conditions are right), we find that there is a specific class of ANOVA designs for which repeated observations are taken on each subject. Not surprisingly, these are called **repeated measures ANOVAs** and are a direct extension of the paired t test.

For example, suppose we repeat the ASA study; only this time, each patient gets to use all six drugs on six successive headaches. To the extent that some folks get more severe headaches and some get less severe headaches, we should find systematic differences between subjects. And if we can account for these differences, we have effectively removed some of the "error" variance in the previous analysis by attributing it to systematic differences between patients, leaving less in the error term. This should increase

Table 5-4
ANOVA Table for Cold Reliever Study

Source	Sum of Squares	Degrees of Freedom	Mean Square	F	p
RN/HC	112.5	1	112.5	4.10	< 0.05
BS/SP	112.5	1	112.5	4.10	< 0.05
BS/SP $\times$ RN/HC	112.5	1	112.5	4.10	< 0.05
Brand	125.0	2	62.5	2.27	NS
Brand $\times$ RN/HC	512.5	2	256.25	9.33	< 0.001
Error	5,270.0	192	27.45	—	—

the power of the statistical test of brands, just as a paired *t* test increased the power of the *t* test.

Suppose we re-arrange the previous data set (see Table 5-1) in order to recognize that it was actually the same patients in all six groups. The data might now look like Table 5-5.

Note that these are the same data. The means for each drug are exactly the same. However, this time, we have included the means for each patient (which we couldn't do before because there were 20 patients with only one rating each). Now the ANOVA table looks like Table 5-6.

You'll see that the Sum of Squares due to drug is exactly the same as before (80.00), and so is the total Sum of Squares (140.00). This tells you that we did use the same data as before. However, we have accounted for a lot of the remaining Sum of Squares by differences between subjects (53.67), leaving much less in the error term. And the statistical test for drug has increased from an *F* of 6.4 to an *F* of 42.38!

From where did the Sum of Squares due to subjects come? By a direct extension of what we have been doing all along, taking the differences between individual subjects' means (eg, 6.17, 7.00), subtracting the grand mean (8.0), and squaring the whole lot. (This whole sum has to be multiplied by the number of drugs, six, to get the right answer.)

The net result, in this case, is to add a lot to the statistical power by removing variance due to subjects, just as we gained power with the paired *t* test. We also economized on subjects although more was asked of each one.

Table 5-5
Pain Ratings for Five Patients and Six Pain Relievers

	Drug						
Patient	**A**	**B**	**C**	**D**	**E**	**F**	**Mean**
1	5	6	7	9	4	6	6.17
2	6	8	8	10	5	5	7.00
3	7	7	9	11	6	7	7.83
4	8	9	11	12	7	9	9.33
5	9	10	10	13	8	8	9.67
Mean	7.0	8.0	9.0	11.0	6.0	7.0	—

Table 5-6
ANOVA Table Treating Drugs as a Repeated Factor

Source	Sum of Squares	Degrees of Freedom	Mean Square	*F*	Tail Prob
Subjects	53.67	4	13.42	42.38	< 0.0001
Drugs	80.00	5	16.00	50.53	< 0.0001
Error	6.33	20	0.32	—	—

This is the simplest of repeated measures ANOVA designs. Of course, we can extend it to multiple factors. For example, suppose the first three subjects were stoic women and the last two were snivelling men. We could introduce a new "between subjects" factor, sex, and add a few more lines to the ANOVA table, which would now look like Table 5-7.

Now we have a main effect of sex (mean square = 45.00), which actually accounted for much of the differences between subjects in the previous analysis. We have a Drug × Sex interaction, which turns out to be zero, indicating that the two sexes respond equally well to individual drugs.

This time, there was no gain in statistical power. Why? Because we have lost 5 degrees of freedom in the error term, resulting from the extra means we had to estimate, so the mean square actually went up a bit. If there had been a Drug × Sex interaction, there might still have been a gain in power because this would explain some of the variance in response to individual drugs.

Two important lessons can be learned: (1) the complexity of research designs for ANOVA is limited only to the imagination of the investigator and the stamina of the subjects, and (2) there is a law of diminishing returns, whereby the additional variance explained is negated by the loss of degrees of freedom.

As you can appreciate, the technique is a powerful one, albeit a little mysterious. You can now, without committing any statistical atrocities, consider an experiment that tests several hypotheses simultaneously, and you can look at how different factors interact with each other. The example we have chosen is one of a semi-infinite number of possibilities, limited only by the imagination. Some of these variations are catalogued. For example, **repeated measures ANOVA** is used if we take several measures on each subject by letting each subject try each reliever in succession. Other specific design terms include **Latin square, split-plot, fractional factorial**, and on and on, the specifics of which go far beyond our present needs.

But factorial ANOVA has some disadvantages. Conceptually, it is still the familiar game of comparing variation due to differences between group

Table 5-7
ANOVA Table Adding the Effect of Sex

Source	Sum of Squares	Degrees of Freedom	Mean Square	F	Tail Prob
Sex	45.00	1	45.00	15.58	< 0.05
Error (between)	8.67	3	2.88	—	—
Drugs	76.80	5	15.36	36.38	< 0.0001
Drugs × Sex	0.00	5	0.00	0.00	1.00
Error (within)	6.33	15	0.42	—	—

means to variation of individual values within groups; however, by the time you get to four or five factors, the results can become uninterpretable because the differences are buried in a mass of three-way and four-way interaction terms. Also, the assumptions of ANOVA are more stringent than those for the z test or for the t test, and this tends to be forgotten by many experimenters. In particular, the standard deviations within each cell of the design must be approximately equal. The design must be balanced, that is to say, there must be an equal number of subjects in each cell, or you cannot directly interpret the main effects and interactions.

C.R.A.P. DETECTORS

Example 5-1

A study compared three different antacids for relief of gastric pain. The dependent variable was the pH of gastric contents after treatment. Twenty subjects, 10 men and 10 women, were in each group. A t test showed that C was better than A ($p < 0.05$) and better than B ($p < 0.001$), but there was no difference between A and B.

Question. Can you improve on the analysis?

Answer. First, the comparison of the three groups is just begging for a one-way ANOVA. However, if you use sex as a second factor, systematic differences between men and women may emerge, as well as interactions. Finally, p values notwithstanding, the author has left us with no idea of the magnitude of the effect.

C.R.A.P. Detector V-1

Generally, there are more errors committed in not using ANOVA than in using it. Multiple comparisons demand ANOVA.

C.R.A.P. Detector V-2

Don't be misled by all the F ratios. Authors should still provide means and standard deviations so you can tell the magnitude of the effect.

C.R.A.P. Detector V-3

Generally, the use of multiple factors, which splits up the total variance among several independent variables, results in a smaller error term and a more powerful test.

6

Relationship between Interval and Ratio Variables: Linear and Multiple Regression

> *Regression analysis* deals with the situation in which there is one measured dependent variable and one or more measured independent variables. The *Pearson correlation* and the *multiple correlation coefficients* describe the strength of the relationship between the variables.

$Despite\ the\ fact$ that you have been introduced to some statistical sledgehammers in the last few chapters, you might have noticed that the conditions under which they could be applied were somewhat restrictive. One variable was always a nominal variable (eg, reader–nonreader, clam juice–no clam juice), and the other variable was always interval or ratio. Although that fairly well describes the situation in many studies, there are two other combinations that frequently arise. The first is when both variables are nominal or ordinal (eg, dead–alive, cured–not cured), in which case we must use **nonparametric statistics**. This situation will be dealt with in Part 3.

The second class of studies are those in which both independent variables (IVs) and dependent variables (DVs) are interval or ratio. This situation frequently arises when the researcher cannot institute an experiment in which some people get it and some don't. Instead, the experimenter must deal with natural variation in the real world, in which people may, of their own volition, acquire varying degrees of something and then have more or less of the DV.

For example, suppose you want to examine the relationship between obesity and blood sugar. In the best of all possible worlds, you would take a sample of newborn infants and randomize them into two groups. Group A members would be raised on puréed pizza, milk shakes, and potato chips for the next 40 years, and Group B members would have small quantities of rabbit food during the same period. But the ethics committee wouldn't like it, and the granting agency wouldn't fund it. So a more likely approach would be to venture timorously out into the real world, grab a bunch of complacent and compliant folks, measure their skinfold and blood sugar, and plot a graph depicting the relationship between them. If the relationship was really strong, these points would lie on a straight line. Unfortunately, these relationships don't occur often in the real world because there are usually many variables, both known and unknown, that might affect blood sugar. So there is bound to be a great deal of scatter about the average line, and the first challenge may be determining where to draw the line.

If you recall your geometry, you might remember that a straight-line equation is described as follows:

$$\text{Blood sugar} = a + b \times \text{skinfold}$$

The y intercept of the line is "a," and the slope is "b." The issue, then, is "What combination of "a" and "b" yields the best fit?"

The way statisticians approach this is to define "best" in a particular way. As shown in Figure 6-1, they determine the vertical distances between the original data ($\cdot$) and the corresponding points on the line ($\bigcirc$), square these distances, and sum over all the data points. They then select a value of "a" and "b" that results in the least value for this sum, called a **least squares criterion**. This Sum of Squares, which is an expression of the deviation of individual data from the best-fitted line, is exactly analogous to the Sum of Squares (within) in an analysis of variance (ANOVA) and is called the **Sum of Squares (residual)**. A second Sum of Squares can then be calculated by taking the differences between the points on the line and the horizontal line through the two means, squaring, and adding. This one is analogous to the Sum of Squares (between) in ANOVA and is called the **Sum of Squares due to regression**.

TESTING SIGNIFICANCE AND STRENGTH OF RELATIONSHIP IN SIMPLE REGRESSION

Although you can do a test of significance on the Pearson correlation (see p. 58) to determine if there is a relationship between the IVs and DVs, this significance testing commonly comes about in a different way. Frequently, the computer printout will list a table of numbers with headings like those in Table 6-1. The coefficients are the intercept (constant), which equals 98.0 and can be identified on the graph. Similarly, the second line of the table is the slope of the regression line, which equals 1.14. The computer also

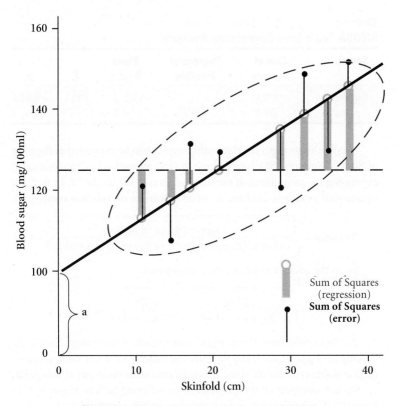

Figure 6-1 Relationship between blood sugar and skinfold.

calculates the standard error (SE) of these estimates, using complicated formulas. The t test is the coefficient divided by its SE, with $n - 2$ degrees of freedom (where n is the sample size), and the significance level follows.

Usually, the computer also prints out an "ANOVA table." But, sez you,
"I thought we were doing regression, not ANOVA." We have already drawn
the parallel between regression and ANOVA in the previous section. These
Sums of Squares end up in the ANOVA table as shown in Table 6-2. If you
take the square root of the F ratio, it equals exactly the t value calculated earlier (as it should because it is testing the same relationship).

Table 6-1
Output from Regression Analysis

Variable	Coefficient	SE	t	Significance
Constant	98.00	12.3	7.97	0.0001
Skinfold	1.14	0.046	24.70	0.0001

SE = standard error.

Table 6-2

ANOVA Table from Regression Analysis

Source	Sum of Squares	Degrees of Freedom	Mean Square	F	p
Regression	2,401.5	1	2,401.5	610.1	< 0.0001
Residual	270.0	18	15.0	—	—

Finally, the strength of relationship could then be expressed as the ratio of Sum of Squares (SS) (regression) to [SS (regression) + SS (residual)], expressing the proportion of variance accounted for by the IV. In fact, the square root usually is used and is called a **Pearson correlation coefficient**.

$$\text{Correlation} = \sqrt{\frac{\text{Sum of Squares (regression)}}{\text{Sum of Squares (regression)} + \text{Sum of Squares (residual)}}}$$

So, in the present example, the correlation is:

$$R = \sqrt{\frac{\text{SS (reg)}}{\text{SS (reg)} + \text{SS (res)}}} = \sqrt{\frac{2,401.5}{2,401.5 + 270.0}} = 0.95$$

We also could have tested significance of the relationship directly by looking up significance levels for different values of the correlation coefficient and different sample sizes. This is, of course, unnecessary at this point.

We can interpret all this graphically by referring back to Figure 6-1. In general, the individual data points constitute an ellipse around the fitted line. The correlation coefficient is related to the length and width of the ellipse. A higher correlation is associated with a thinner ellipse and better agreement between actual and predicted values.

TWO OR MORE INDEPENDENT VARIABLES: MULTIPLE REGRESSION

In the previous example, we dealt with the relationship between blood sugar and skinfold. This is the simplest form of regression analysis in that there is one IV, one DV, and a presumed straight-line relationship between the two. A bit of reflection suggests that blood sugar is likely to be influenced by other variables, diet and heredity, for example. If these could be used, it seems likely that our ability to predict blood sugar levels would improve. There is a fair amount of mileage to be gained by using several IVs in predicting a DV. The technique is called **multiple regression** and is an extension of the previous approach.

Suppose, for example, you are chair of the admissions committee for the residency training program in pediatric gerontology at Mount Vesuvius Hospital. Every year, you have interviewed all the applicants to the program, but you wonder if you might save some money and predict performance better by using previous academic records. Performance in the program is based on a rating by supervisors. The academic record of applicants contains (1) grade point average in medical school (MDGPA), (2) National Board license examination (NBE) results, and (3) undergraduate grade point average (UGPA). The regression equation using these IVs might look like the following:

$$\text{Performance} = a + (b \times \text{MDGPA}) + (c \times \text{NBE}) + (d \times \text{UGPA})$$

The statistical analysis is conducted by estimating values of the parameters $a \rightarrow d$ in such a way as to minimize the squared differences between the real data and the estimated points. Essentially, what the computer is doing is fitting a straight line in four-dimensional space (you will forgive us if we don't include a figure). And once again, the overall goodness of fit is determined by calculating a correlation coefficient from the ratio of the variance fitted by the line to the total variance. This correlation coefficient is called the **multiple correlation** (symbolized as R). The square of the multiple correlation can be interpreted directly as the proportion of the variance in the DV (ratings, in this example) accounted for by the IVs.

Of course, that isn't all the information obtained from the analysis. The computer also estimates the coefficients a to d and does significance testing on each one. These coefficients indicate the degree of relationship between performance and each IV after the effects of all other variables have been accounted for.

Suppose, for example, that the resultant regression equation looked like the following:

$$\text{Performance} = 0.5 \times (0.9 \times \text{MDGPA}) + (0.04 \times \text{NBE}) + (0.1 \times \text{UGPA})$$

The estimated coefficients (0.9, 0.04, 0.1) are called **unstandardized regression coefficients** (funny name, because they look standard enough). It would appear that MDGPA predicts quite a bit, and NBE, very little. But let's take a closer look. Suppose MDGPAs have a mean of 3.5 and a standard deviation (SD) of 0.25. Then a change of one SD in MDGPA results in a change of $0.9 \times 0.25 = 0.225$ in performance. By contrast, if NBE scores have a mean of 75% and SD of 20%, a change of one SD yields a change in performance of $20 \times 0.04 = 0.8$ units in performance. So the size of the coefficient doesn't reveal directly how predictive the variable is. To make life easier, we often transform these to **standardized regression coefficients** or **beta weights** by converting each variable to have a mean of 0 and SD of 1. The resulting weights can then be compared directly. In the present example, that would result in weights of 0.53 for NBE results and 0.15 for MDGPA; thus, NBE result is approximately three times as strong a predictor as MDGPA.

You might have your interest piqued by these results to explore the situation a bit further. For example, if you can do nearly as well without the UGPA, you might be prepared to forgo this requirement. The question you now wish to ask is "How much do I gain in prediction by adding in UGPA?"

One approach to this question would be to fit another regression line, using only MDGPA and NBE scores and determining the multiple correlation. The difference between the squared multiple correlations for the two equations, with UGPA in and out of the prediction, tells you how much additional variance you have accounted for by including the variable. This is the basic process in **stepwise regression**, a method whereby predictor variables are introduced one at a time into the regression equation and the change in the multiple correlation is determined. There are two ways of approaching stepwise regression: either you can introduce the variables into the equation in some logical order specified by the experimenter, as in the current example, or you can let the computer decide the sequence.

The computer method is probably more popular. There are a number of esoteric criteria used to determine the order in which variables will be introduced. Basically, the computer enters them in an order of decreasing ability to account for additional variances, a sort of statistical law of diminishing returns, so that at some point, you can determine at what point little is to be gained by adding more predictor variables. The cutoff can be based on the statistical consideration that the contribution of an additional variable is not statistically significant. Alternatively, it can rest on more pragmatic grounds, namely, that the additional explained variance isn't worth the effort.

Although stepwise regression in which the computer does all the work is likely more popular because it avoids any deep thought on the part of the researcher, it has fallen on hard times at the hands of real statisticians. The reason, of course, is a statistical one.

To understand this, put yourself in the shoes of a computer—something that is lightning fast but kind of thick (like some of the guys on athletic scholarships). You are doing stepwise regression on someone's pet database consisting of 193 variables on 211 subjects. You have searched the data for the most significant relationship and have put it into the equation. Now it's time to find the next one, which you do by doing a whole bunch of new regression analyses with two variables in the equation, recalculating all the significance levels as if each of the remaining 191 variables were lucky enough to be chosen. That's 191 F tests. You put the lucky variable in the equation next, then repeat the procedure to find the next variable—another 190 significance tests.

The big trouble is that some of those significant F tests got that way by chance alone, based on random variation in the data set. The chances of replicating the findings with a new database are the same as that of a snowball's survival in Arizona in July. The solution is to go back to the old way, entering the variables according to a sequence laid out in advance by the experimenter. It's more intellectually satisfying, too. You can enter variables systematically according to a theory (eg, family structure "causes" family dysfunction "causing" loss of self esteem, which, with life stress, "causes" depression) or on more pragmatic grounds (in the above example, MDGPA is more standardized and relevant than UGPA). To ensure that everybody knows you're still doing science, you can glorify the whole process with a big term: **hierarchical regression**.

Carrying the analysis of our example one step further, the data from the regression analysis might be presented in the style of Table 6-3. The data show each step of the analysis on each successive line. The first step is just a simple regression, with the multiple R^2 equal to the square of the simple correlation $(0.50)^2 = 0.25$. The computer then calculated an F ratio, which proved to be statistically significant. At the second step, MDGPA was added, explaining an additional 8% of the variance, and again, this was statistically significant. Finally, introducing UGPA explained only 2% more of the variance and was not significant.

One bit of subtlety: sometimes, a variable that has a high simple correlation with the DV won't do anything in the multiple regression equation. Returning to our blood sugar example, an alternative measure of obesity might be kilograms above ideal weight, and it might correlate with blood sugar nearly as well as skinfold. But it's likely that the two are highly correlated, so if skinfold goes into the regression equation first, it is probable that kilograms won't explain much additional variance and may not be significant.

The message here is that a variable may not be a useful predictor of the DV, for two reasons. First, it has a low correlation with the DV. Second, it has a reasonable correlation with the DV but is highly correlated with another IV that has higher correlation with the DV and enters the equation first.

So that's what multiple regression looks like. Beware the study founded on a large database but with no prior hypotheses to test with an adequate experimental design. The investigators can hardly resist the temptation to bring out the statistical heavy artillery such as multiple regression to reach

Table 6-3
Results of Stepwise Regression Predicting Resident Performance

Step	Variable	Multiple R^2	Change in R^2	F Ratio	Significance
1	NBE score	0.25	—	13.78	< 0.0001
2	MDGPA	0.33	0.08	3.02	< 0.05
3	UGPA	0.35	0.02	1.78	NS

MDGPA = medical school grade point average; NBE = National Board examination; NS = not significant; R = multiple correlation; UGPA = undergraduate grade point average.

complex, glorious, and often unjustified conclusions about the relationships between variables.

C.R.A.P. DETECTORS

Example 6-1

A large database gathered during a 10-year period in a certain Midwestern town ($n = 12,498$) was analyzed to determine predictors of high serum cholesterol. Twenty-eight different dietary factors were examined, and it was found that serum calcium levels correlated -0.07 ($p < 0.05$) with serum cholesterol levels. The investigators concluded that low calcium causes high cholesterol.

Question. Will you drink more milk?

Answer. Not from these findings. A correlation of -0.07 is statistically significant because of the large sample, but it accounts for only $0.07^2 = 0.49\%$ of the variance. Anyway, we would expect that one of the 28 variables would be significant by chance alone. Finally, the association may be caused by something else.

C.R.A.P. Detector VI-1

Beware the large sample, revisited. With large samples, statistical significance loses all relationship to clinical significance.

C.R.A.P. Detector VI-2

Watch out for fishing expeditions. The meaning of $p < 0.05$ applies equally well to correlation coefficients.

C.R.A.P. Detector VI-3

Correlation does not imply causation. Height and weight are highly correlated, but height doesn't *cause* weight. Researchers can get carried away when they see large correlations and can start to interpret them as evidence of a causal relationship.

Example 6-2

A teacher of dyslexic children interviewed the parents of 12 of his students and found that birth order was significantly correlated with reading test scores ($R = 0.65$, $p < 0.05$). He concluded that lack of parent stimulation in infancy, which is more likely in large families, is a cause of reading problems.

Question. Do you agree?

Answer. There are a few difficulties here. With only 12 kids, one or two from very large families could bump up a correlation, significance notwith-standing. Also, the fact that birth order was correlated with dyslexia does not imply a causative relationship.

C.R.A.P. Detector VI-4

Beware the small sample, revisited. It is easy to obtain correlations that are impressively large but cannot be replicated. A good rule of thumb is that the *sample size, or number of data points, should be at least five times the number of IVs.*

C.R.A.P. Detector VI-5

Regression equations may fit a set of data quite well. But extrapolating beyond the initial data set to values higher or lower is tenuous.

C.R.A.P. Detector VI-6

The multiple correlation is only an indicator of how well the initial data were fit by the regression model. If the model is used for different data, the fit won't be as good because of statistical fluctuations in the initial data.

7

Analysis of Covariance

> Analysis of covariance combines both regression and analysis of variance. There is one measured dependent variable. However, the independent variables can be both categorical factors and measured variables.

In the past few chapters we have developed a number of ways to analyze continuous data. *Factorial analysis of variance* deals nicely with the problem of nominal independent variables (IVs) or factors, and *multiple regression* techniques deal with the case of several continuous predictor variables. All looks to be in fine shape.

Unfortunately, experiments in the real world are not so neatly categorized as these two techniques might suggest. A number of situations can arise in which the IVs may be a mixture of categorical and continuous variables, which cannot be dealt with adequately by either analysis of variance (ANOVA) or regression techniques, such as when investigators are doing the following:

1. Examining the relative effectiveness of several drugs on subjective ratings of angina, adjusting for the degree of narrowing of coronary arteries, as measured by angiography
2. Determining the relationship between dietary iron and hemoglobin levels, controlling for sex
3. Predicting the severity of arthritis measured by the number of affected joints, from laboratory data, including sedimentation rate (millimeters per hour) and rheumatoid factor (+/−)

In each of these situations, the dependent variable (DV) is continuous with interval data, but the IVs are a combination of nominal and interval data. A statistical method that combines the best of both ANOVA and regression techniques is required. There are two approaches to dealing with this class of problems: **analysis of covariance (ANCOVA)** and the **general linear model (GLM)** (more on the GLM in Chapter 8).

Suppose a psychiatrist decides to add one more study to the growing number of studies that contrast one mode of psychotherapy with another. The two most popular methods of treating depression in middle age (Tired Yuppie Syndrome [TYS]), are Primal Scream (PS) and Hot Tub Hydrotherapy (HTH); the outcome measure will be length of time in therapy. If the psychiatrist left it at this, things would be straightforward: assemble a group of blue yuppies, randomize to HTH or PS, count weeks in therapy, and do a *t* test on the means. But it is evident that his patients come in all shades of depression, from light blue to deep purple, and this is likely to affect outcome. So a better approach is to measure the degree of depression, using a standard scale, before starting therapy.

Now if HTH actually worked better than PS, resulting in fewer weeks of therapy, a plot of the DV against the initial depression scores might look like the one depicted in Figure 7-1. The slope of the two lines indicates a linear

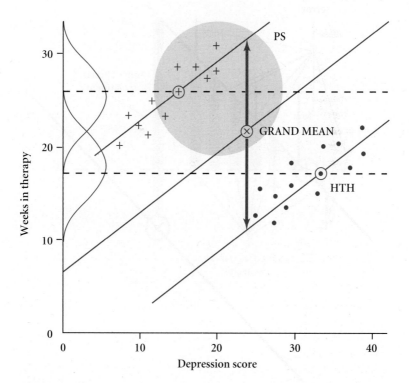

Figure 7-1 Relationship between initial depression score, treatment modality, and time in treatment.

relationship between degree of depression and time in therapy, and the vertical distance between the two lines is the relative effect of the two therapies. Finally, the error of the prediction is measured by the dispersion of individual points from the two lines.

ANCOVA proceeds to fit the data with two lines, just as in regression analysis, estimating the slope of the lines and the difference between them. Statistical significance is tested by breaking the total variation in the data into the following three components (Figure 7-2):

1. **Sum of Squares due to regression (now called a covariate).** This corresponds to the difference between the points on the fitted line and the corresponding horizontal line through the group mean. This is completely analogous to the regression case.

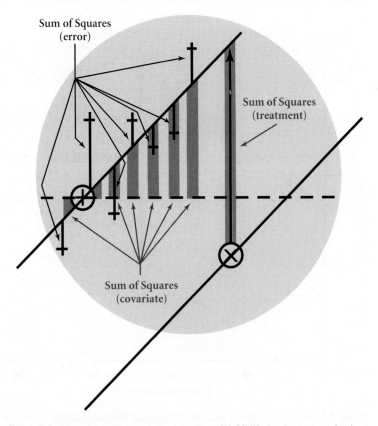

Figure 7-2 Enlarged view of an analysis of covariance (ANCOVA), showing sources of variance.

2. **Sum of Squares due to treatments.** This is based on the difference between the means in each group, and the grand mean, analogous to ANOVA.

3. **Sum of Squares due to error.** Just as with regression and ANOVA, this is merely the difference between the original data and fitted points.

Then, by playing around with degrees of freedom and mean squares, we can develop *F* ratios to determine whether each effect is significant. The results are displayed in a table similar to an ANOVA table, except there is an additional line for the covariate.

Note what happens when all the data are projected onto the *y* axis (see Figure 7-1), which would be the case if the data were simply analyzed with ANOVA. First, because mean depression scores differed in the groups, the projected means are much closer together, leading to an underestimate of the size of the difference between two groups. Second, the dispersion of the data around the group means has increased by a factor of two or three. So a statistical test based simply on the differences between the group means could be biased and would be much less likely to detect a difference between groups than ANCOVA. Turning it around, the potential advantages of ANCOVA are an increase in precision (hence, an increase in the power to detect differences) and an ability to compensate for initial differences in the two groups.

However, this potential gain can be realized only if there is a relationship between the dependent measure and the covariate, and the gain in precision is related directly to the strength of the relationship. Taking the extreme cases, if the correlation between the covariate and the dependent measure were 1.0, then all the data would lie on the two lines. There would be no error variance, and the statistical test of the difference between treatments would be infinite. Conversely, if there were absolutely no relationships between the two measures, the two lines would be horizontal, the situation would be identical to projecting the data on the *y* axis, and the investigator would have simply expended a lot of effort—and more importantly, a degree of freedom—to no avail.

It is a usual requirement that there is *no* relationship between the experimental treatment (the grouping factor) and the covariate, which would amount to different slopes in each group. The reason for this condition is that if there was a relationship, it would not be possible to sort out the effects of covariate and treatment because the treatment effect would be different for each value of the covariate. This possible confounding is usually prevented by measuring the covariate before implementing the treatment.

The basic approach can be extended to multiple covariates and multiple factors in the design, limited only by the imagination and the size of the data processing budget. However, similar issues apply to the choice of covariates as predictive variables in regression analysis. Ideally, each covariate should be highly correlated with the DV but independent of each other covariate. This provides a practical limitation to the numbers of covariates that are likely to be useful.

C.R.A.P. DETECTORS

Example 7-1

A psychologist got into a verbal exchange with a colleague about two modes of behavior therapy for patients with photonumerophobia.* He likes a gradual increase in exposure to the noxious stimulus whereas his buddy throws his patients into the deep end and then gives lots of support. To resolve the issue, they do a study in which the DV is galvanic skin response, an index of anxiety, measured while subjects are delivering a research paper. After the lecture, subjects are then asked to recall how anxious they were before treatment by using a rating scale, to be used as a covariable. The covariate was significant ($p < 0.05$), but no treatment differences were found.

*Fear that their fear of numbers will come to light.

Question. Who wins the bet?

Answer. No one. Because the covariate was measured after treatment, people who responded well may rate their initial anxiety lower than those who didn't respond. Then, if one method worked better, the final anxiety in this group would be lower, but so would the initial anxiety, leading to an underestimate of the treatment effect.

C.R.A.P. Detector VII-1

Take a close look at when and how the covariate was measured, and reassure yourself that it could not be confounded with the grouping variables.

C.R.A.P. Detector VII-2

No amount of ANCOVA can safely adjust for initial differences between groups. Random allocation is better by far.

C.R.A.P. Detector VII-3

Look closely at the size of the mean square of the covariate. If it's small, assume the researchers are just trying to dazzle you with statistical shotguns and don't know what they're doing.

8

Variations on Linear Regression: Logistic Regression, General Linear Model, and Hierarchical Linear Models

Linear regression is the basis of a number of advanced methods: logistic regression, when the dependent variable is dichotomous; the general linear model, which allows both continuous and categorical independent variables; and hierarchical linear models, when the parameter estimates are themselves random variables.

LOGISTIC REGRESSION

When we looked at multiple regression, we dealt with the situation in which we had a slew of independent variables that we wanted to use to predict a continuous dependent variable (DV). Sometimes, though, we want to predict a DV that has only two states, such as dead or alive, or pregnant versus not pregnant. If we coded the DV as 0 for one state and 1 for the other and threw this into a multiple regression, we'd end up in some cases with predicted values that were greater than 1 or less than 0. Statisticians (and real people, too) have difficulty interpreting answers that say that some people are better than alive or worse than dead. So they had to come up with a way to *constrain* the answer to be between 0 and 1, and the method was **logistic regression**.

Let's start off by setting the scene. Several years ago, when my daughter was still at home, she taught me more about 1960s rock music than I (Geoffrey Norman) ever knew in the '60s. I grew to recognize the Steve

Miller Band, Pink Floyd, Led Zeppelin, Jefferson Airplane, and the Rolling Stones. (I was okay on the Beatles and on the Mamas and the Papas, honest!) The intervening years have been unkind to rock stars. Buddy Holly, the Big Bopper, and Richie Valens were the first to go, in a plane crash way back then. Hendrix, Jim Morrison, Janis Joplin, and Mama Cass all went young, mostly to drugs. Elvis succumbed to a profligate excess of everything. Nasty diseases got Zappa and George Harrison, and Lennon met an untimely death outside the Dakota Hotel in Manhattan. Indeed, at one point, I commented to my daughter that all her heroes were 5 years older than me or had pegged off two decades before she was born.

Why is the risk of death so high for rock stars? Lifestyle, of course, comes to mind. Hard drugs take their toll, as do too many late nights with too much booze. Travel in small planes from one gig to the next is another risk. Celebrity has its risks. (In passing, the riskiest peacetime occupation we know is not that of lumberjack or miner—it's that of president of the United States. Four of 43 US presidents have been assassinated, and four have died in office—not to mention those who were brain-dead before entering office—for a fatality rate of 18.6%.)

Suppose we wanted to put it together and assemble a Rock Risk Ratio, or R^3—a prediction of the chances of a rock star's dying prematurely, based on lifestyle factors. We assemble a long list of rock stars, present and past, dead and alive, and determine what lifestyle factors might have contributed to the demise of some of them. Some possibilities are shown in Table 8-1.

Now, if R^3 were a continuous variable, we would have a situation in which we're trying to predict it from a bunch of continuous and discrete variables. As we mentioned, that's a job for multiple regression. We would just make up a regression equation to predict R^3 from a combination of DRUG, BOOZE, CONC, and GRAM, like this:

$$R^3 = b_0 = b_1 \text{ DRUG} + b_2 \text{ BOOZE} + b_3 \text{ GRAM} + b_4 \text{ CONC}$$

The trouble is that death is not continuous (although aging makes it feel that way); it's just 1 or 0, dead or alive. But the equation would dump out some number that could potentially go from $-$infinity to $+$ infinity. We could re-interpret it as some index on some arbitrary scale of being dead or alive, but that's not so good because the starting data are still 0s and 1s, and that's

Table 8-1
Lifestyle Factors Contributing to the Demise of Rock Stars

Variable	Description	Type	Values
DRUG	Hard drug use	Nominal	Yes / No
BOOZ	Excess alcohol use	Nominal	Yes / No
GRAM	Number of Grammies	Interval	0 – 20
CONC	Average no. of live concerts / year	Interval	0 – 50

what we're trying to fit. It would be nice if we could interpret these fitted numbers as probabilities, but probabilities don't go in a straight line forever; they are bounded by 0 and 1 whereas our fitted data don't have these bounds.

Maybe, with a bit of subterfuge, we could get around the problem by transforming things so that the expression for R^3 ranges smoothly only between 0 and 1. One such transformation is the **logistic** transformation:

$$p\,(\text{DEAD}\,|R^3) = \frac{1}{1 + e^{-R^3}}$$

Looks complicated, huh? (For our Canadian colleagues, "Looks complicated, eh?") Keep in mind that what we have here is the probability of dying at a given value of R^3. If you remember some high school math, when $R^3 = 0$, p is $1\,/\,(1 + \exp(\infty)) = 1\,/\,(1 + 1) = 0.5$. When R^3 goes to infinity (∞), it becomes $1\,/\,(1 + \exp\text{-}(\infty)) = 1$, and when R^3 goes to $-\infty$, it becomes $1\,/\,(1 + \exp(\infty)) = 0$. So it describes a smooth curve that approaches 0 for large negative values of R^3, goes to 1 when R^3 is large and positive, and is 0.5 when R^3 is 0. A graph of the resulting **logistic equation** is shown in Figure 8-1.

So when the risk factors together give you a large negative value of R^3, your chance of dying is near zero; when they give you a large positive value, up your life insurance because the probability gets near 1.

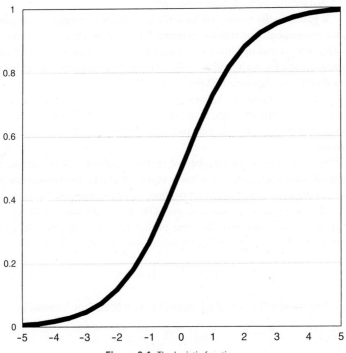

Figure 8-1 The logistic function.

So far, so good. But all the risk factors are now buried in the middle of a messy equation. However, with some chicanery, which we will spare you, we can make it all look a bit better:

$$\log \frac{p}{1 - p} = (b_0 + b_1 \text{ DRUG} + b_2 \text{ BOOZE} + b_3 \text{ GRAM} + b_4 \text{ CONC})$$

Lo and behold, the linear regression is back (except that the expression on the left looks a bit strange). But there is a subtle difference. We're computing some continuous expression from the combination of risk factors, but what we're predicting is still 1 or 0. So the error in the prediction amounts to the difference between the predicted value of $\log [p / (1 - p)]$ and 1 if the singer in question has croaked or between $\log [p / (1 - p)]$ and 0 if he or she is still alive.

The issue now is how we actually compute the coefficients. In ordinary regression, we calculate things in such a way as to minimize the summed squared error (called the **method of least squares**). For arcane reasons, that's a no-no here. Instead, we must use an alternative and computationally intensive method called **maximum likelihood estimation** (**MLE**). Why you use this is of interest only to real statisticians, so present company (you and we) are exempt from having to undergo explanation. Suffice it to say that at the end, we have a set of parameters, the bs, with associated significance tests, just like we did with multiple regression.

If you have the misfortune of actually doing the analysis, you might, to your amazement, find that the printout is not too weird. Just as in multiple regression, we end up with a list of coefficients and their standard errors, a statistical test for each, and a p value. However, usually, the last column is another left hook, labeled ***EXP(b)***.

A cautionary note: the next bit involves some high school algebra around exponents and logs. If you don't remember this arcane stuff, either go read about it or skip the next paragraph. Likely, you'll be no worse off at the end.

So here we go. What's happening is this: we began with something that had all the b coefficients in a linear equation inside an exponential; now we're working backwards to that original equation. Suppose the only variable that was predictive was drug use (DRUG), which has only two values, 1 (present) or 0 (absent). Now the probability of death, given drug use, means that DRUG = 1, and the equation looks like the following:

$$\log \left[\frac{p_1}{(1 - p_1)} \right] = b_0 + b_1$$

And if there is no drug use, then DRUG = 0, and the formula is:

$$\log \left[\frac{p_0}{(1 - p_0)} \right] = b_0$$

If we subtract the second from the first, then we get the difference between the two logs on the left, and b_1, all by itself, on the right. But the difference between logs is the log of the ratio. So we end up with the following:

$$\log\left[\frac{p_1/(1-p_1)}{}\right] = b_1$$

And as a final step, we get rid of the logs and end up with:

$$\frac{p_1(1-p_1)}{} = e^{b_1}$$

Now the ratio $p/(1-p)$ is an **odds** (see p. 105), so that mysterious last column, *EXP(b)*, is just the **odds ratio**. So, for example, if the coefficient for DRUG was 2.5, then $e^{+2.5} = 12.18$, and the odds of the rock star's dying if he did drugs is 12.18 when compared to drug-free rock stars (both of them).

Another thing that is commonly done with logistic regression is to see how well it did in predicting eventual status (which is easy if you wait long enough). All you do is call all predicted probabilities of 0.49999 or less a prediction of ALIVE, and of 0.5 or greater a prediction of DEAD, then compare the prediction to the truth in a 2 × 2 table. There are also statistical tests of goodness of fit related to the likelihood function, tests on which you can put a *p* value if the mood strikes you. *

In summary, logistic regression analysis is a powerful extension of multiple regression for use when the dependent variable is categorical (0 and 1). It works by computing a logistic function from the predictor variables and then comparing the computed probabilities to the 1s and 0s.

THE GENERAL LINEAR MODEL

When we learned statistics, one of the mantras we were taught to mumble, as we searched for inner peace, was "ANOVA (analysis of variance) and regression are just subsets of the general linear model." Then, just when it looked like analysis of covariance (ANCOVA) was the ideal general method, someone noted that it was also a special case and that there was a more general way of looking at things, which in turn was called the **general linear model (GLM)**. At the time, we had no idea what it actually meant, but it sounded profound and dazzled them at frat parties. Indeed, when we wrote the first and second editions of *PDQ Statistics*, we still didn't know, and we passed off the explanation as being much too complicated for our dear readers. Well, we finally figured it out. So here goes!

Let's go back to the ANCOVA example we used in the previous chapter for a moment. We had two groups, Hot Tub Hydrotherapy (HTH) and Primal Scream (PS), and we were using depression score as a covariate.

Suppose we forget, for the moment, that HTH versus PS is a categorical variable and just create a regression equation with these two independent variables to predict the number of weeks of therapy:

$$\text{Weeks} = a + b \times \text{Depression} + c \times \text{HTH/PS}$$

Now let's do a little diddling, called creating a **dummy variable** (no doubt referring to the deluded folks who were silly enough to sign up for these treatments). If someone is in the HTH group, we'll score this variable as a 0, and if they're in the PS group, we'll give them a 1. This has the effect of creating two parallel regression lines, one for the HTH group:

$$\text{Weeks} = a + b \times \text{Depression} + c \times 0 = a + b \times \text{Depression}$$

and one for the PS group:

$$\text{Weeks} = a + b \times \text{Depression} + c \times 1 = (a + c) + b \times \text{Depression}$$

So the overall effect of the PS treatment compared to HTH is just the constant term, c, added on. And if we do a multiple regression, it will treat this dummy variable like any other, estimate it (giving us an estimate of the treatment effect), and do significance tests on it (giving us the needed p value).

As it happens, nothing in the multiple regression theory says that the *independent* variables have to be interval, normally distributed, or anything else. And working through the example like this will yield *exactly the same results* as the ANCOVA. So what we've done is turn the whole thing into one very general linear model—*the* general linear model.

The GLM has some advantages over ANCOVA. We needn't worry about interaction terms between treatments and covariates; we can model them with additional terms in the equation. We also don't have to worry about having equal sample sizes in every group, a constant worry of those doing complicated ANOVAs.

Frequently Asked Question 1. Why is it called the general linear model?

Because (at least until structural equation models came along—we'll discuss these later) it was the most general type of equation. With it, you could do everything from a simple t test through ANOVA and ANCOVA, multiple regression, and even canonical correlation and discriminant function analysis (we'll also discuss these later).

Frequently Asked Question 2. Why don't we do GLM all the time?

In the old pre-PC days, before Pentium 4s and gigabyte hard drives, people had to actually calculate these ruddy things by hand. Because GLM was harder to calculate, it was the method of last resort. Today, it is a bit harder to set up than ANOVA or regression, but there is really no other reason. Like many other statistical tests, ANCOVA exists for computational simplicity, nothing more. In fact, most computer programs give you options like ANOVA, ANCOVA, or regression as a front end, but all are actually doing a GLM analysis deep in their bowels.

HIERARCHICAL LINEAR MODELS

For all the regression stuff we've done up until now, the dependent variable still involves only one observation per subject. We have no equivalent to the paired *t* test or repeated measures ANOVA, in which we take many observations (typically over time) on each case. It's time to rectify this egregious oversight.

Let's think for a moment about a lifetime of booze consumption. We are not passing judgment in doing so; unlike the prohibitionists, we prefer to point out that moderate drinking, particularly of red wine at an average of two glasses per day, apparently confers a health benefit, to the tune of a 10% reduction in overall mortality—far better, we might point out, than cholesterol-lowering drugs (although apparently ethanol is one, and certainly one of the most pleasant, at that). A small hooker is that those concerned with alcohol consumption regard the same two glasses a day as borderline alcoholism in North America (although in Europe, it's probably five glasses per day, and in Russia, we imagine that anything less than five bottles of vodka a day is viewed as abstaining).

Anyway, how would we go about studying it? We could imagine identifying a cohort of perhaps 500 16-year-olds and then following them at, say, 5-year intervals for the next 50 years (we can't imagine us doing it, though). When they reach age 65 years or so, we call off the study and start analyzing. Now if these were all compliant folks, they would dutifully show up on our doorstep every 5 years on the nose; they would not move away, get committed, go to prison, or die; and after 50 years, we would have a nice data set of 11 observations on 500 people. We could go blithely on and do a repeated measures ANOVA on everyone. No problem!

Actually, there are several problems. The first is one of interpretation. After we do the ANOVA, all we'll have to show for it is a significant or non-significant effect of time, telling us whether average booze consumption changes with age. But that's not what we want to know; we're really looking for *how* it changes with age, not *if* it changes. In ANOVA, the independent variable or factor is treated as a nominal variable—just a bunch of categories. As far as the analysis is concerned, these categories are completely interchangeable, with no implied order. We get the same answer if we rearrange the time periods. The result is that if there's any time trend, such as a linear improvement, we'll never know about it.

The solution to this is actually simple. We push the "orthogonal decomposition" button on the big blue machine, and it will tell us whether there's a linear trend, a quadratic trend, etc, all the way up to a term for the power of 10 (one less than the number of observations). The computer assumes that the categories are successive observations over time with equal spacing and fits a straight line, then a quadratic function, and so on, to the data. At least now we know how things are changing on average over time.

Now to the next problem. That's how the *average* person progresses. But in this game, no one is average. Some try a few drinks, then quit altogether. Some go overboard, head for a fall, and then go on the wagon, only to cycle again. Some start low and stay low. Some gradually increase consumption with each decade. Is there any way, we ask, to capture this individual variation in change over time?

A related question has a practical bent to it. Inevitably, some subjects die young by car accident, some miss appointments with the researcher in favor of appointments with the prison system, some arrive a year or two late, and others drop out altogether or move away or whatever. The rub is that with any missing observation, ANOVA drops the whole case, so pretty soon we have no study subjects at all. Yet, from the perspective of looking at each individual or at the group, missing observations are not that big a crisis in that they don't preclude plotting the curve over time. In fact, even the simple case in which one person showed up only on even assessment points and another on odd points is enough to send ANOVA into spasms and leave us with no cases although we would have a lot of data to figure out how both of them change over time.

Let's reformulate the whole problem as a regression problem. In fact, let's reformulate it as a series of regression problems, one for each subject. Each line will have an intercept, b_0, and a slope, b_1 (the linear term); then we can throw in higher-order terms, such as $time^2$, $time^3$, $time^4$, and so on, up to as many powers as we have points, minus 1. The general equation would be of the following form:

$$\text{Booze/week} = b_0 + b_1\,\text{Time} + b_2\,\text{Time}^2 + b_3\,\text{Time}^3 + \ldots\, b_{(n-1)}\,\text{Time}^{n-1}$$

Consider a few cases. Subject 1 starts drinking at age 16 years at two snorts a week and stays that way until he's 65 years old. He's just a straight horizontal line (in regression terms, that is). The second guy starts at one snort per week, and every 5 years, he increases his drinking by two. For him, $b_0 = 1$, $b_1 = 2$, and b_2 through $b_{(n-1)} = 0$. A third sad case just gets worse and worse and ends up in the gutter—$b_0 = 1$, $b_1 = 2$, $b_2 = 3$, and the rest $= 0$. And so it goes. For each case, we can draw a regression line through the points (regardless of where in time these are actually measured). What we have then determined is called an **individual growth curve**.

And now the supreme subterfuge. We're still interested in the overall trend, so what we now do is treat all the *b*s as data. Instead of looking at the original data on booze consumption, we now just look at the calculated b_0, b_1, b_2, etc., for each subject and treat them as the raw data, distributed normally with a mean and a standard deviation. So the mean of the b_0s is the average consumption at 16 years of age, the mean of the b_1s is the average change in consumption over a 5-year period, and so on. We can go on and do significance tests on these computed parameters, just as in ordinary regression.

Then comes a final twist. We can go to the next step and ask questions such as "What factors make a guy turn to the devil booze, and what factors protect him from the evils of liquor?" Essentially, what we are saying is "Can we predict the slope of the booze/time curve for each individual?" For example, maybe a disrupted childhood leads to social isolation. So we predict each guy's slope by using measures of number of moves, divorce of parents, childhood friends, and so forth—another regression equation, only the input for this regression equation is the output from the last one (the b_1s for each subject in the sample). What we have created is a hierarchy of regression equations. You would think that we might call it "hierarchical regression." Unfortunately, that term is already taken, so instead, we call it (using the newfound wisdom of a few pages earlier) a **hierarchical linear model (HLM)**.

Actually, that wasn't the final twist; there's one more. Let's say that we now turn our attention to what determines how kids do in school. As with any study, we gather a host of variables about each kid, starting with grades and also throwing in stuff about the education of the parents, the number of books in the home, and the amount of time the kid spends watching television. But we know (from sometimes painful experience) that the kids' performance is also affected by their teachers and by the atmosphere in the school itself, so we also get data about these. The problem is that the teacher factors apply to 20 or 30 kids and that the school ones apply to 50 or so teachers and a few hundred kids. One way to handle this is with ANOVA, with kids **nested** within teacher and with teacher nested within school; but then we wouldn't be able to use the regression equation at the level of the kids. A more elegant way is to use HLMs: the "lowest" level involves the kids, the next highest level applies to teachers, and the top level looks at the schools. In this way, we can determine the influence of the school on the teachers and the teachers on the kids, and we can then look at the factors affecting the kids themselves. Complicated, but it answers all of the questions.

In summary, HLM approaches are a godsend for longitudinal data, where inevitably some people miss appointments, some die or move away, and some arrive a week or a month late. We are no longer locked into a fixed schedule of observations and a complete data set. Further, you can actually get at the question that matters, namely, how people change over time, individually and together. There is one cautionary note: while it is easy to assume that dropouts, missed appointments, and other mishaps occur at random, they likely don't. The people who miss appointments are, by definition, different from those who don't, and no amount of statistical gimcrackery will compensate for this (see Chapter 20). So some caution should be exercised if there are too many missing data. The technique is also useful·(nay, required) when there are "hierarchies" of effects.

C.R.A.P. DETECTORS

Example 8-1

To examine the impact of invasive procedures on quality of life, a researcher identifies a group of patients with abdominal pain. She administers a quality-of-life questionnaire to both groups and then does the following: (a) she follows up the patients to see who undergoes endoscopy and who has no procedure done, and (b) she also asks each patient to complete a symptom diary for 10 days and calculates the proportion of days that the patient had symptoms.

Question. How would you analyze (a) and (b)?

Answer. This is a trick question. Although it looks like (a) could be a logistic regression with quality-of-life predicting the likelihood of getting endoscopy, all you need after the dust settles is a t test on the quality-of-life score, with endoscopy/none as the grouping factor. Action (b) is analyzed the same way because although the dependent variable is a proportion, it is actually an interval level variable. You only analyze it with nonparametric statistics when the datum on each person is a 1 or a 0.

C.R.A.P. Detector VIII-1

Sometimes, the independent and dependent variables for analysis are the opposite of what might be assumed based on consideration of cause and effect.

C.R.A.P. Detector VIII-2

You use logistic regression and the like when the outcome for each individual is binary, not when the data are proportions.

Example 8-2

A researcher starts off to do a longitudinal study of depression with stage 3 breast cancer patients. His particular interest is how depression changes over time after diagnosis. He administers the Beck Depression Inventory at the time of initial diagnosis and every 3 months for the next 2 years. He begins with 150 patients, but has only 84 left by 2 years. He asks you to run a repeated measures ANOVA on the 84 survivors.

Question. Any ideas of what to tell him?

Answer. "Get lost and leave me alone" immediately comes to mind. Obviously, the 84 patients who are still around differ systematically from the 126 poor lost souls. They have one good reason to be less depressed—they're still here!

Still, assuming many of those who died were alive long enough to observe over several follow-up visits, even if not over all eight visits, you might be able to come up with some useful data by doing an individual growth curve analysis and looking at the curves of the survivors and the deceased. You could, within the HLM approach, actually do a significance test on the various coefficients for survivors versus deceased to see whether there is a significant difference.

C.R.A.P. Detector VIII-3

Individual growth curve analysis works very well for longitudinal data with missing values. However, it must be used intelligently, as in this analysis, which explicitly recognizes the differences between those who survived and those who did not.

9

Time Series Analysis

Time series analysis allows us to look at data where we make many repeated measurements on the same individual or organization over time. Because each value is correlated with the preceding and following data points to some degree, some special problems arise.

A *topic closely associated* with multiple regression is **time series analysis** (**TSA**). Both techniques attempt to fit a line (most often, a straight one) to a series of data points. However, whereas multiple regression analysis (MRA) examines how various independent variables (IVs) operate together to produce an effect, TSA looks at changes in one variable over time. We do this in an informal and nonstatistical way every day. For example, in deciding whether or not to wear a coat today, we review the trend in the temperature over the past few days; or before investing the $20,000 we have just lying around gathering dust, we look at the performance of the stock market in general or of a specific company over the last few months. (We should note that some people rely on this "informal time series analysis" in situations where it shouldn't be used. After seeing four reds in a row at the roulette wheel, they bet more heavily on black, erroneously assuming that its probability of occurrence is dependent on the previous spins. This is called the "gambler's fallacy," and its perpetuation is fervently prayed for each night by casino owners.)

Although these examples may seem reasonable to a meteorologist or an economist, we rarely simply examine trends over time. More often, we are interested in somewhat different questions: Did things change after some *intervention*? Did the rate of automobile deaths fall after the speed limit was reduced? Was there a higher incidence of Guillain-Barré syndrome after the swine flu vaccination program was begun? Did the emptying of the psychiatric hospitals follow or precede the introduction of phenothiazines? The technical term for this line of questioning is *interrupted time series analysis* because it examines the effects of an intervention that may interrupt the ongoing pattern of events. The traditional way of representing this is

O O O O O X O O O O O

where the Os are observations of some variable over time and where X represents the intervention. (We could, of course, use an "I" for the intervention, but this would be too logical.) This shows that we have two sets of observations, those made before the intervention and those made after it. Observations can be of a single person or event over time (eg, the price of a certain stock during 1 year or a child's behavior in a classroom during the semester), or each observation can consist of the mean of different people or events (eg, looking at how successive classes of applicants score on the Medical College Admission Test).

These examples point to two major differences between MRA and TSA. First, in MRA, we are looking at the relationship between one dependent variable (DV) and one or more IVs; in TSA, the interest is in changes in a single variable over time. The second difference, and one of significant consequence, is that in TSA, the data are **serially correlated**. What this very impressive term means is that the value of the variable at time 1 is related to and affects the value at time 2, which in turn is related to and affects the time 3 value. For example, today's temperature is dependent in part on yesterday's; it may differ by a few degrees one way or the other, but a large variation would be unexpected. Moreover, this implies that the **temporal order** of the variables is important; generally, the value for time 5 must fall between those of time 4 and time 6 to make sense of the trend. Multiple regression is not designed to handle this serial dependency, so it should not be used to analyze time series data although this has never stopped people from misapplying it in the past and most likely will not stop them from doing so in the future.

When we are looking for the effects of some intervention, we can ask three questions: (1) Has the *level* of the variable changed? (2) Has the *rate of change* of the variable changed? (3) Have *both* the level and rate of change of the variable changed?*

The easiest way to explain what these questions mean is through a few examples. To begin with, let's assume that we've just heard of a new golf ball that is guaranteed to shave five strokes from our game. How can we check this out? One way would be to play one game with our old ball, then play one with the new ball, and compare scores. However, we know that the scores

---

*There are also a number of other questions we can ask, such as, "Was the change immediate, or was there a delay?" "Did the change occur gradually or suddenly?" "Did it have a permanent effect or only a temporary one?" In fact, TSA can probably tell you more about the data than you really want to know.

vary from day to day, depending in part on how we're feeling but also because of our improvement (we hope) over time. So any "positive" result with the second ball could be the result of a combination of natural fluctuations in our score, coupled with our expected improvement. What we need, therefore, is to play enough games with the first ball so that we have a *stable* estimate of our score, then play enough rounds with the second ball to be confident we know our new average score. Figure 9-1 illustrates the variability in scores for the first six games played with the old ball and the latter six games played with the new ball. The arrow indicates when the intervention took place and where we would expect to see an interruption in the time series. Our question would be, "Taking into account our slow improvement over time and the variability in the two sets of scores, is the *level* of our scores lower, the same, or higher after the change?" Naturally, if there is a constant increase or decrease in the level of the scores, the average of the preintervention scores will always be different from the postintervention average. So when we talk about a "change in level," we compare the last preintervention score with the first one after the interruption. Before we tell you how we figure this out, we'll give a few more examples.

Despite what the drug manufacturers would like us to believe, there's some evidence that psychiatric hospitals began emptying out before the introduction of the major tranquilizers in 1955. If this is true, then we cannot simply look at the hospital census in 1954 and compare it with the 1956 census because the decrease may be due to something other than drugs. Our

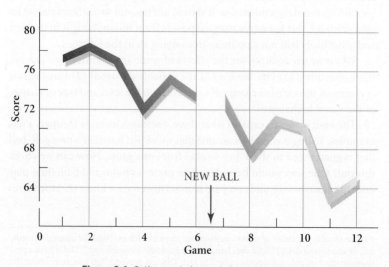

Figure 9-1 Golf scores before and after using a new ball.

question has to be a bit more sophisticated: did the *rate* of emptying change because of the introduction of psychotropic medications? We can begin by plotting the total number of patients in psychiatric beds in the 10 years prior to our time of interest and for the following 10 years, as shown in Figure 9-2 (don't believe the actual numbers; they were made up for this graph). Let's examine some possible outcomes. In Figure 9-2, (a), it appears as if the intervention has had no effect; neither the slope nor the level of the line has changed following the introduction of the new medication. In (b), there has been a sudden drop in the level, but the slope remains the same. This can occur if a large number of people are suddenly discharged at one time but the steady outflow of patients is unchanged. For example, it's possible that over the time span examined, the hospitals had begun keeping acute patients for shorter periods of time, accounting for the sudden drop, but that this did not hasten (or slow down) the steady discharge of other patients. In (c), a situation is shown in which the rate of discharge of patients was speeded up by the new drug but without a mass discharge of patients at one time. Last, (d) shows both effects happening at once (ie, a sudden discharge of patients followed by an increased discharge rate for the remaining patients). These are not the only possible patterns; let your imagination run wild and see how many others you can dream up. Try adding a delayed effect, a temporary effect, a gradual effect, and so on.

Let's turn our attention from *what* TSA does to how it achieves such miracles. One factor that makes interpreting the graph more difficult is that the value of the variable may change over time, even without any intervention. If the change is always in one direction, it is called a **trend**. A gradual change one way followed by a gradual change the other way is referred to as **drift**. If we have relatively few data points, it may be difficult to differentiate between the two. The primary cause of trend or drift is the dependency of a value at one point on previous values. As we mentioned before, this is called **serial dependency**, and we find out if it exists by calculating the **autocorrelation coefficient**. When we compute a normal run-of-the-mill correlation, we have two sets of scores, X and Y, and the result can tell us how well we can predict one from the other. The "pairs" of scores are formed somewhat differently in autocorrelations; the value at time 1 is paired with the value at time 2, time 2 is paired with time 3, and so on. In a way analogous to a Pearson correlation, this tells us to what degree scores at time t are predictive of scores at time $t + 1$, and this is referred to as a **lag 1 autocorrelation**. However, the effect at time t may be powerful enough to affect scores down the line. We can explore this by lagging the scores by two units (eg, time 1 with time 3, time 2 with time 4), three units (time 1 with time 4, time 2 with time 5), and so forth. If the lag 1 autocorrelation is significant (ie, if the data are serially dependent), then the autocorrelations most often become smaller as the lags get larger. This makes sense on an intuitive level because the effect of one event on subsequent ones usually dissipates over time.

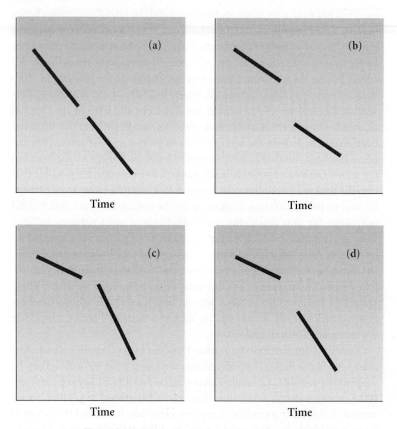

Figure 9-2 Different possible results from an intervention.

A significant autocorrelation can be due to one of two causes: the scores themselves may be serially correlated, or sudden "shocks" to the system may have effects that last over time. The first situation is called the **autoregression model** whereas the second is referred to as the **moving averages model**. Thus, this is known as the **autoregressive integrated moving averages** (**ARIMA**) technique. Moving averages is another trick statisticians use to smooth out a messy line; that is, one with fluctuations from one observation to the next. We can take the average of scores 1 and 2, then the average of 2 and 3, then of 3 and 4, and so on. If the curve hasn't been smoothed enough, we increase the *order* of smoothing, by averaging scores 1, 2, and 3; then scores 2, 3, and 4; then 4, 5, and 6, etc, until the end of the series. Since the extreme score is "diluted" by averaging it with more "normal" scores, its effect is thereby lessened. Theoretically, we can continue this until we have only one number, the mean of all the scores.

Our next step is to try to remove the effect of the trend or drift in order to see if there is any change in the level. This is done by **differencing** the time series, which means that the observation at time 1 is subtracted from the one at time 2, the time 2 observation is subtracted from the time 3 observation, and so forth. Let's see how this works. Assume we have the following sequence of numbers:

1 3 5 7 9 11 13

If we were to draw these on a graph, a definite trend would be apparent since the points would increase in value with every observation period. Now, let's take the **differences** between adjacent pairs of numbers. What we get is

2 2 2 2 2 2

So it's obvious that there is no trend; the line is flat over all the observations. Note two things: first, there is one less differenced number than original observations, and second and more importantly, life is never this beautiful or clean-cut.

The success of differencing is checked by recalculating the autocorrelation. If it works, then the autocorrelation should quickly (ie, after a few lags) drop to zero, and the series is said to be **stationary**. If there is still a trend, we repeat the process by subtracting the first differenced value from the second, the second from the third, and so on. Although in theory we can repeat this process of autocorrelating and differencing many times (or at least until we run out of numbers because we lose one observation each time we difference), we need only do it once or twice in practice.

Up to this point, what TSA has done is to try to determine what factors can account for the data. This is done by going through the following sequence of steps:

1. Compute the lagged autocorrelations to determine if the sequence is *stationary* or *nonstationary*.

2. If the sequence is nonstationary, *difference* the scores until it becomes stationary.

3. Recompute the autocorrelations to see if the trend or drift is due to an *autoregressive* or a *moving averages* process.

These steps are referred to collectively as *model identification*. The next stages involve actually trying out this model with the data to see how well they fit. This involves estimating various parameters in the model and then diagnosing any discrepancies. Again, this is an interactive process since any discrepancies suggest that we have to identify a new model, estimate new parameters, and again diagnose the results.

Once all this is done we can move on to the last step, which is to see if the intervention had any effect. One way of doing this is simply to analyze the preintervention and postintervention data separately and then to compare the two models. The parameters will tell us if there has been a change in the trend, in the level, or in both. We are fortunate that computer programs exist to do the work for us although this is a mixed blessing because it has allowed people to analyze inappropriate data and report results that best belong in the garbage pail.

C.R.A.P. DETECTORS

Example 9-1

It has been suggested that even brief psychotherapy can reduce medical utilization. To test this out, a researcher looks at the total dollar expenditure on health care in a group of patients for each of the 12-month periods before and after therapy.

Question 1. Can these data be analyzed with TSA?

Answer. The *type* of data are appropriate for TSA, but there are too few data points. In order to get a stable estimate of the parameters, the researcher should have at least 30 (yes, 30) observations in each set. Lately, there seems to be a contest on to see who can analyze the sequence with the fewest number of points. This is an extremely unfortunate trend (pardon the pun) because this technique clearly is inappropriate with fewer than 30 observations, especially if there are wide fluctuations from one point to another.

C.R.A.P. Detector IX-1

In TSA, look for at least 30 preintervention and postintervention measurements.

Question 2. The researcher's conclusions read simply, "A time series analysis showed significant changes after a course of therapy." What's missing?

Answer. What model did the researcher use? Autoregressive? Moving averages? Another? With so many options, the researcher must tell us what assumptions were made before we can accept the conclusions drawn by statistical methods.

C.R.A.P. Detector IX-2

If the author does not state whether or not the data were differenced or whether an autoregressive or a moving averages model was used, don't bother reading further. If the model was specified, the author must give the reasons for using one model rather than another.

Part Three

Nonparametric Statistics

10

Nonparametric Tests of Significance

A variety of statistical tests have been devised to examine the association between a single categorical independent variable (IV) and nominal or ordinal dependent variables (DVs). These include the *chi-square test*, the *binominal test*, and *Fisher's exact test* for nominal data and independent samples; the *McNemar chi-square test* for related samples; the *Mann-Whitney U, median, Kruskal-Wallis*, and *Kolmogorov-Smirnov* tests for ordinal data and independent samples; and the *sign test* and *Wilcoxon test* for ordinal data and matched samples.

A*lthough quantitative measurement* is essential to the biologic disciplines that are the basis of the health sciences, clinical research is often more concerned with the practical issues of preventing disease, treating illness, and prolonging life. The object of measurement, in turn, is determining the presence or absence of risk factors, assessing the presence or absence of particular diseases, and estimating survival (the presence or absence of death). These measures are all nominal categories, and the numbers are body counts (eg, the number of people with angina, treated with a β-blocker, who survived 1 year). These kinds of data require different kinds of statistical methods, called **nonparametric statistics**, for analysis. By far the most common nonparametric test is the **chi-square test**.

TESTS FOR NOMINAL DATA

The Chi-Square Test

There has been a great deal of discussion about the possible adverse health effects of video display terminals (VDTs). Because this book was written on a VDT, the question is of more than passing interest. One factor that clouds the issue, however, is that the people who are most exposed to VDTs are also in pressure cooker jobs; so stress, not radiation, may be the real problem. To put it to the test, let's examine a different form of VDT, the kind that populates video arcades and is strictly for recreation. Because the adverse health effects seem to be rare, we might go for a case-control design: first locate a group of young mothers who experienced complications of pregnancy, then compare them, on the basis of time spent in video arcades during pregnancy, with a group of mothers who had normal deliveries. The data might look like those arrayed in Table 10-1.

If exposure had no effect, we would expect that the proportion of individuals in both groups who had been in arcades to be the same. The best guess of this proportion is based on the sum of both groups, 110/300 or 36.7%. So the expected number exposed in the cases is just 0.367 × 100 or 36.7, and the control group is 0.367 × 200 = 73.3. Similarly, the expected frequencies in the bottom two cells are 63.3 and 126.7.

One way to test the statistical significance of the association is to determine the difference between the observed and expected frequencies and to proceed to create a variance term, as we've done many times before, by squaring the differences and adding them up:

$$(60 - 36.7)^2 + (50 - 73.3)^2 + (40 - 63.3)^2 + (150 - 126.7)^2$$

Now the usual approach would be to go looking for some way to estimate the standard error (SE) of the differences to use as a denominator. In contrast to our previous examples, we don't have any individual values in each cell to estimate the standard deviation (SD), just a single number. But fortunately, Mother Nature comes to the rescue. It turns out that as long as

Table 10-1
Association of Pregnancy Complications in Young Women and Exposure to Video Display Terminals in Video Arcades

Exposure	Complicated Pregnancy	Normal Pregnancy	Total
Yes	60	50	110
No	40	150	190
Total	100	200	300

the expected frequencies are fairly large, they are normally distributed, with a variance equal to the frequency itself. For an expected frequency of 16, the variance is 16 and the SD is 4. Because the variance is simply the expected frequency in each cell, the approach is to divide each term separately by its expected frequency. The test looks like this:

$$\frac{(60-36.7)^2}{36.7} + \frac{(50-73.3)^2}{73.3} + \frac{(40-63.3)^2}{63.3} + \frac{(150-126.7)^2}{126.7} = 35.17$$

This ratio is called **chi-square** (χ^2), by far the most commonly used non-parametric test. The larger its value, the more the numbers in the table differ from those we would expect if there were no association. So the chi-square test is a test of the association between two variables. It can easily be extended to more than two levels for each variable. For example, we could have defined time in the video arcades as high, low, or none, resulting in a 2×3 table.

The bad news is that χ^2 has a few limitations. The first is that it assumes no ordering among the categories but treats the categorical variable as nominal. That's okay if it is a nominal variable, but if the categories are ordered, there's information that isn't being used by the test. A second problem is that when the expected frequency in any cell is small—less than 5 or so—the test is inaccurate.

The two alternatives that can be used with analyses that have small expected frequencies are both based on calculating the exact probability that the particular frequencies that were observed could have occurred by chance. Both tests yield exact answers, even when frequencies in some cells are zero, but they can be applied only under very restricted circumstances.

The Binomial Test

The binomial test is a one-sample test, like the z test in parametric statistics. In addition, it is restricted to only two cells.

Suppose we had six patients with a very rare disease, Tanganyikan restaurant syndrome. Detailed statistics collected by the previous British Raj indicate a survival rate of 50%. After a course of therapy consisting of puréed granola and wild bee honey, five patients remain alive. Is this a statistically significant improvement in survival?

If the expected survival rate is 50%, then the likelihood that any one patient would survive is 0.5; so the probability that all six patients would survive is $0.5^6 = 1/64$. With a little more probability logic, we can see that there are six ways that five of the six patients would survive: patient 1 dies and the rest live, patient 2 dies and the rest live, and so on. The probability of any one outcome is still 0.5^6, so the probability of five survivors is $6 \times 0.5^6 = 6/64$. Since we are trying to reject the null hypothesis, we want to determine the likelihood that five survivors or any more extreme numbers could arise by chance if the expected number of survivors were 50%, or three. Thus, the overall probability of five or more survivors, under the null hypothesis, is 6/64 + 1/64 = 7/64, which is not significant. So we would conclude, in this example, that there has not been a significant decrease in fatality rate.

The approach can be extended to other expected probabilities by some fancier formulas, but the approach of adding up the exact probability of the observed and all more extreme possibilities remains the same.

That's the binomial test. Again, a reminder that the binomial test is a useful replacement for χ^2 when the expected frequencies are less than five, but it only works for a single sample with two cells.

Fisher's Exact Test

The equivalent exact test to the binomial test for the case of two independent samples is Fisher's exact test. Like the binomial test, Fisher's exact test is a useful replacement for χ^2 when the expected frequencies are small, and only two responses are possible. A common situation in which Fisher's exact test must be used is in the analysis of trials in which the outcome of interest (such as death) occurs fairly infrequently.

Since there is some suggestive evidence that alcohol may reduce the rate of heart disease, how about a trial in which half the folks get vodka with their orange juice and half don't? Five years later, we look at cardiac deaths and see the results in Table 10-2.

The null hypothesis is that there is no difference in the proportion of deaths in the two groups. A chi-square test cannot be used because the expected frequencies in the two bottom cells are too small (ie, 5.5), so it's necessary to use an exact test. A complicated formula from probability theory exists to calculate the exact probability.

To see where it comes from, imagine that the Grim Reapress is sitting across the bar from the drinkers. She sees 200 drinkers knocking back screwdrivers and decides that it's time to take one out. She randomly aims her cardiac bullet at one person. How many choices does she have for the first boozer? Answer: 200. Now it's time to remove another one. How many

Table 10-2
Comparison of Cardiac Death Rates of Vodka Drinkers and Nondrinkers

	Vodka Drinkers	**Control**	**Total**
Alive	197	192	389
Dead	3	8	11
Total	200	200	400

possibilities? Answer: 199, of course; one is already lying in a heap on the barroom floor. And for the last of the drinkers: 198.

So the number of ways three imbibers could have been taken out by fate is 200 × 199 × 198. But there's another wrinkle. Once they're gone, neither we nor the grieving relatives really care about the order in which they met their demise, so we have to see how many ways we could have ordered three bodies on the barroom floor. Three could have ended up on the bottom of the pile. Once this is decided, two could have been in the middle, and now there is only one choice for the top of the pile. So as to the number of ways to drop 3 boozers from 200, the answer is:

$$\text{Number of ways} = \frac{200 \times 199 \times 198}{} = 1{,}313{,}400$$

A shorthand way to write this is with factorials ($10! = 10 \times 9 \times 8 \times 7 \times 6 \times 5 \times 4 \times 3 \times 2 \times 1$). So the preceding formula is:

$$\text{Number of ways} = \frac{200!}{3! \ 197!} = 1{,}313{,}400$$

By the same logic, the number of ways eight teetotalers could have dropped is:

$$\text{Number of ways} = \frac{200!}{8! \ 192!} = 55 \times 10^{12}$$

However, we are looking for association. So we have to ask, what is the probability that you could have gotten eight dead on one side and three on the other? To answer this, we have to work out the number of ways that 11 people out of 400 could have died, regardless of their drinking habits. This works the same way:

$$\text{Number of ways} = \frac{400!}{11! \ 389!}, \text{ which is a huge number.}$$

Finally, the probability that all this could have worked out the way it did is:

$$\frac{\dfrac{200!}{8! \ 192!} \times \dfrac{200!}{3! \ 197!}}{\dfrac{400!}{11! \ 389!}}$$

After some cross-multiplying, this equals:

$$\frac{200! \times 200! \times 11! \times 389!}{400! \times 3! \times 8! \times 197! \times 192!} = 0.161$$

Table 10-3
Effect of Vodka Consumption on Cardiac Death Frequency

	Vodka Drinkers	Controls	Vodka Drinkers	Controls	Vodka Drinkers	Controls
Alive	198	191	199	190	200	189
Dead	2	9	1	10	0	11

More generally, if you go back to the original table, you can see that the formula is:

$$\frac{(a + b)!\ (a + c)!\ (b + d)!\ (c + d)!}{N!\ a!\ b!\ c!\ d!}$$

where a, b, c, and d are the numbers in the top left, top right, bottom left, and bottom right cells, and N is the total.

But to test the null hypothesis, you also have to determine the probability of all the more extreme values. To get at the more extreme values, you keep the marginal values fixed (keep the totals of each row and column [ie, 200, 200, 389, and 11] the same) and reduce the value in the smallest cell by one until it is zero. In our example, the more extreme values, keeping the same marginals, are shown in Table 10-3.

It's simply a case of sticking these three combinations into the formula (which determines the probability of occurrence of each combination by chance), adding up the probabilities, and concluding whether the total probability is sufficiently small to reject the null hypothesis. In case you're interested, by our calculations these probabilities are, respectively, 0.051, 0.012, and 0.002. So the total probability is:

$$p = 0.161 + 0.052 + 0.012 + 0.002 = 0.227$$

This may provide comfort and solace to drinkers and teetotalers alike.

The McNemar Test

As the chi-square test and Fisher's exact test are to the unpaired *t* test, so the McNemar test is to the paired *t* test. It is used for two related measures on the same sample or for other situations in which each individual measurement in one sample can be paired with a particular measurement in the other. The ordinary chi-square test assumes independence of sampling in the two groups and therefore cannot be used at all when the two samples are matched. The McNemar test is a modification of χ^2 that takes into account the matching of the samples.

As we write this section, we are immersed in yet another election campaign. As usual, both major political parties are assaulting the voters' senses with television commercials showing the candidate—every hair in place, pearly white teeth gleaming—surrounded by equally handsome happy people and delivering with gusto the message that either (1) the economy has never been better (party in power) or (2) the economy has never been worse (the other party). One wonders whether the ad agency ever bothered trying to find out if these inane bits of fluff could change anyone's mind. It would be easy to do. You could grab 100 folks off the street, find out their political allegiance (if any), inflict the commercial on them, and see if any change has resulted. The data might look like Table 10-4.

Note that the only people on whom the commercial had any effect are those in cells "b" and "c." As a result of the commercial, 15 people changed from donkeys to elephants, and 10 changed the other way. It is these cells on which we will focus.

Under the null hypothesis of no effect, we would expect that as many people would change in one direction as the other; that is to say, the expected value of each cell is:

$$\frac{(b+c)}{2} = \frac{25}{2} = 12.5$$

From here on in, it's easy. We simply use the observed values in the changed cells and these expected values, in a chi-square calculation:

$$\chi^2 = \frac{(15 - 12.5)^2}{12.5} + \frac{(10 - 12.5)^2}{12.5} = 1.0$$

This is distributed, more or less, as a chi-square distribution with one degree of freedom. It turns out that a better approximation to chi-square, for mysterious reasons, is determined by subtracting one from the numerator; after some algebra, we get:

$$\chi^2 = \frac{[(b-c)-1]^2}{(b+c)} = \frac{[(15-10)-1]^2}{25} = 0.64$$

Compare the χ^2 value with the table to determine significance, and that's the McNemar test. Since the value was not significant, we would conclude that neither was the commercial.

Table 10-4
Effect of Television Commercial on Party Allegiance

	Donkey	Elephant
Before	35[a]	15[b]
After	10[c]	40[d]

NONPARAMETRIC TESTS ON ORDINAL VARIABLES

In previous chapters, we have made the point that the use of nonparametric tests on data that are interval or ratio is akin to throwing away information. Similarly, applying a test such as the chi-square test to data that can be ordered can also result in a loss of information.

A wide variety of nonparametric tests can be applied to this situation. For some bizarre reason, nearly all of these tests were developed by two-person teams, unlike the one-person shows of Fisher, Pearson, and Student. In this section, we're going to have a look at a series of partnership efforts: Mann and Whitney, Kolmogorov and Smirnov, and Kruskal and Wallis.

As an example, let's use the old favorite of pain researchers, the visual analog scale (VAS). The scale is a 10-cm line with labels such as "depressed and near death" at one end and "happy and healthy" at the other. The patient simply puts an "X" on the line indicating how he or she feels. As usual, the title does much to make the method look more sophisticated than it is. Even though you can measure a score to a millimeter or so, there really is no assurance that the psychological distance between 9 cm and "healthy" (10 cm) is the same as that between "death" (0 cm) and 1 cm, so there is some reason to treat these data as ordinal. (The same comments apply to nearly any rating scale if you want to be hard-nosed about it.)

Judging from the commercials, hemorrhoids produce the kind of pain amenable to do-it-yourself solutions. How about a trial of Preparation Help (H) and Preparation P (P), a placebo? We mail one tube of either preparation to 20 of our suffering friends so that 10 receive H and 10 receive P, along with a VAS to fill out. The data might look like Table 10-5.

Table 10-5
Pain Scores for Hemorrhoid Preparations

| | H | | | P | |
Subject	Score	Rank	Subject	Score	Rank
1	9.8	1	11	8.6	5
2	9.6	2	12	8.2	7
3	8.9	3	13	7.7	9
4	8.8	4	14	7.5	10
5	8.4	6	15	6.9	12
6	7.9	8	16	6.7	13
7	7.2	11	17	4.9	17
8	5.8	14	18	4.5	18
9	5.5	15	19	3.5	19
10	5.1	16	20	1.5	20

If these were interval data, then we could simply calculate means and SDs, plug them into a formula, and calculate the results, using the usual t test. But if we aren't prepared to assume that the data are interval, then some other approaches are necessary. Most are based on rank-ordering the combined data in one way or another and then performing the gimcrackery on the ranks. We have taken the liberty of adding combined ranks to the table for further use.

The Mann-Whitney *U* Test

The Mann-Whitney U test looks at the relative ranks of subjects in the two groups. By collapsing the ranks of our hemorrhoid trial together and labeling the origin of each subject by H or P, we can write out those data in this form:

Rank	1	2	3	4	5	6	7	8	9	10	11	12	13	14	15	16	17	18	19	20
Group	H	H	H	H	P	H	P	H	P	P	H	P	P	H	H	H	P	P	P	P

Now if H were truly better, most people would give it a higher rank, all of the H's would be on the left, and all the P's would be on the right.

We develop a total score (called U, naturally) from the total number of times H precedes each P. If all H's were ranked more highly, then each P would be preceded by 10 H's. If things were totally interspersed, then each P would have 5 H's above it and 5 below on average. In this case, the first P has 4 H's ahead, adding 4 to the sum. The next P has 5 ahead, and the next has 6. Working this through the lot, the sum comes out as follows:

$$4 + 5 + 6 + 6 + 7 + 7 + 10 + 10 + 10 + 10 = 75$$

We then rush to the appropriate table, which probably kept Mann and Whitney busy at their calculators for years, and look up our figure of 75 to see whether it is big enough to be significant. It turns out that it isn't. There are some additional wrinkles that are introduced if the sample size is very large and if there are tied ranks (ie, two scores exactly the same), but what we have described is the basic U test.

The Median Test

If we went back to our original data, we could determine that the median score of the entire sample of scores was 7.5. It is fairly straightforward to determine how many in each group are above and below the median. The data end up in a 2 × 2 table as shown in Table 10-6.

This can be analyzed in the same manner as any 2 × 2 table, using chi-square or Fisher's exact test. In this case, Fisher's exact test is appropriate since the expected frequencies in all cells are exactly five. As it turns out, the test is not significant.

Table 10-6

2 × 2 Table Comparing Treatment versus Control Data

	H	P	Total
Above median	7	3	10
Below median	3	7	10
Total	10	10	10

It's no surprise that the median test isn't associated with any two-person team. It is a commonsense thing to do if you want to analyze ordinal data with a chi-square statistic, and the only mystery is how the approach managed to achieve sufficient eminence to find a place all by itself in statistics books.

The Kruskal-Wallis One-Way Analysis of Variance by Ranks

As we indicated earlier, one way of straightening out the curves in ordinal data is to convert the original data into ranks. The data in each group would then look like the two rank columns. In our example, if there are differences between H and P, the average rank in the two groups would differ, and we could proceed to analyze the ranks by analysis of variance (ANOVA). It turns out that the use of ranks results in some simplifications in the formulas, so that after the dust settles, the equivalent of an F test becomes:

$$H = \frac{12}{N(N+1)} \times \frac{\text{sum of (total rank in groups)}^2}{\text{number in each group}} - 3(N+1)$$

where N is the total number of observations.

In this example, the total rank of the H's is 80 and of the P's, 130. The formula becomes:

$$H = \frac{12}{20(21)} \times \frac{(80^2 + 130^2)}{10} - 3 \times 21 = 3.57$$

This is distributed as a chi-square with degrees of freedom equal to the number of groups less one. In our example, the probability is between 0.10 and 0.05, nearly significant.

Note also that this test, like the median test, is not restricted to two groups but can be applied to any number of groups. By the way, all three tests are subject to the same limitations of small numbers as is the chi-square test. In the median test, if the expected value in any cell is less than 5 (ie, any group less than 10), then the investigator should analyze the frequencies with Fisher's exact test. In the Kruskal-Wallis test, if any of the sample sizes in a group is less than 5, then you have to go to a special table of exact probabilities.

The Kolmogorov-Smirnov Test

Let's take one last run at this data set. The Kolmogorov-Smirnov test capitalizes on a **cumulative frequency distribution**, a term that may be unfamiliar but that can be easily understood through our example. If we were to classify the raw scores of the two samples in groups such as 5.6–6.90, 6.1–6.5,... 9.6–10.0, then it is straightforward to count the number of subjects in each group who fall in each category (ie, to develop a frequency distribution).

These frequencies can then be converted into a probability distribution by dividing by the sample size in each group, which is 10 in this case. Finally, we can obtain a "cumulative" probability distribution by starting at the lowest score and adding probabilities. This distribution tells you what proportion of the sample fell in and below the category score; thus, 6/10 or 60% of H's had scores below 8.6. The concept is best illustrated by Figure 10-1, which shows the distributions for the two groups. They start at 0 at the far left and eventually accumulate up to 10.0 as scores increase to the right.

The Kolmogorov-Smirnov test focuses on the difference between these cumulative probability distributions. If the P's have a lower score than the H's on average, then their cumulative distribution will rise to 10/10 more rapidly, as is the case in our data. The greater the difference between scores on the average, the greater will be the difference between the two cumulative distributions in any category.

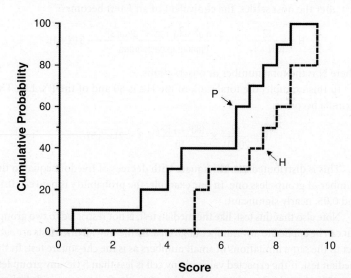

Figure 10-1 Cumulative probability distributions of "H" and "P" groups of hemorrhoid preparation trial.

Now the good news: no fancy calculations or formulas are required to do the Kolmogorov-Smirnov test. All you do is subtract the two probabilities in each category to determine the difference between the two distributions, then find the category with the maximum difference. In our data, that occurs between 4.5 and 5.0 and is a difference of 4/10 or 0.4. That is the value of the Kolmogorov-Smirnov test. And you look in yet another table and find out that the critical value is 0.5, so the difference is not significant.

TESTS OF ORDINAL VARIABLES ON MATCHED SAMPLES

All of the preceding tests on ordinal variables were based on differences among two or more **independent samples** from a population equivalent to an unpaired *t* test in parametric statistics. We have not dealt with the matched or paired situation as yet.

As an example by which to display our wares, suppose a social psychologist predicts that height, since it is one feature of dominance and power, is likely to be associated with success in life. (Before we proceed, we should inform you that one of us is 6 feet 5 inches tall.) In order to cancel out the effect of other environmental variables, such as parents' social class—which might lead on the one hand to better nutrition and greater height and on the other to an "inherited" higher class—the investigator chooses twins of the same sex as subjects. The researcher follows them into adulthood and determines the socioeconomic status (a combination of job class, income, and educational level) of both the taller and the shorter twin.

Suppose the researcher could locate only 10 twins (research grants are hard to come by in the social sciences). The data might look like Table 10-7.

Table 10-7
Sign Test for Correlation of Height and Socioeconomic Status in Twins of the Same Sex

Pair	Taller Twin	Shorter Twin	Differences	Direction
a	87	65	22	+
b	44	40	4	+
c	55	46	9	+
d	69	58	11	+
e	29	16	13	+
f	52	55	−3	−
g	77	60	17	+
h	35	40	−5	−
i	68	50	18	+
j	13	15	−2	−

The Sign Test

The sign test, not surprisingly, focuses on the signs of the differences. If there is no association between height and social status, you would expect that, on the average, half of the signs would be pluses and half would be minuses. The statistical question is, "What is the likelihood that a 7/3 split could occur by chance?" Having reduced the situation to a simple difference between pluses and minuses, the approach is identical to the computational approach we outlined in the binomial test: you calculate the probability of 7 pluses and 3 minuses, 8 pluses and 2 minuses, 9 and 1, and 10 and 0. As it turns out, the probability of obtaining a 7/3 split of pluses and minuses is 0.172, which is not significant.

The Wilcoxon Test

The problem with the sign test, when it is used for ordinal data, is that it ignores the magnitude of the differences. The Wilcoxon test is a bit better in this respect. Let's go back to the data and order it by the magnitude of these differences (Table 10-8).

We're still not allowed to put any direct interpretation on the actual magnitude of the differences, but we can at least say that a difference of 22 is larger than a difference of 18, so the rank ordering of differences has some significance. If there was no relationship between height and status, we would expect that the positive and negative differences would be pretty well intermixed in ranking, and the average rank of positive and negative differences should be about the same.

Table 10-8
Wilcoxon Test for Correlation of Height and Socioeconomic Status in Twins of the Same Sex

Pair	Difference	Rank (+)	Rank (−)
a	22	10	
i	18	9	
g	17	8	
e	13	7	
d	11	6	
c	9	5	
h	−5		4
b	4	3	
f	−3		2
j	−2		1
			7

The Wilcoxon test focuses on these differences in ranks by simply summing the ranks of one sign or another, whichever is ranked lower. In this case, the sum is 7, and if this is located in the appropriate table, the difference is significant at the 0.02 level.

If we blindly assumed that socioeconomic status was interval and calculated a paired t test, the t value would be 2.79, significant at the 0.02 level. So it would appear that the Wilcoxon test, which uses the information about the magnitude of the differences, results in little loss of information in comparison with parametric tests. By contrast, the sign test, which reduces the ordinal data to a plūs or a minus, results in a more conservative test.

DISCUSSION

That's the cookbook of tests that have been applied to ordinal data to test the differences between a sample and theoretical distribution, two samples, or more than two samples. It won't be a surprise to discover that there are a few tests we've left out, such as the Mosteller test of slippage, the K-sample runs test, the randomization test, etc, et al, ad nauseum.

With all these choices, it's a little difficult to make specific recommendations concerning which statistical test to apply and under which circumstances to apply it. In general, the Mann-Whitney and Kruskal-Wallis tests are more powerful, yielding results that are close to parametric tests, and are therefore preferred.

C.R.A.P. DETECTORS

Example 10-1

A naturopath wishes to examine the effect of red iron oxide (rust) supplements on people with anemia. The investigator takes 20 patients, measures their hemoglobin level, and categorizes the disease as mild ($\geq$ 10 g) or severe (< 10 g). Based on clinical information, there were 12 patients with mild disease and 8 patients with severe disease before the study. After the dust settles, there are 16 with mild anemia and 4 with severe. The investigator does a chi-square test on the 2 × 2 table and writes up a study for publication.

Question. There are two boo-boos in the approach; can you spot them?

Answer. First, taking a nice ratio variable such as hemoglobin level and shoving it into two categories is an atrocity. The appropriate test is a paired t test on the differences. Second, these are before–after measurements, so a paired test should be used. If the researcher wanted to categorize, a McNemar test would do. The Wilcoxon test would be the right test for ordinal data.

C.R.A.P. Detector X-1

As we have said many times, classifying ordinal or interval data in nominal categories is throwing away information.

C.R.A.P. Detector X-2

Watch out for small expected frequencies. Exact tests should be used if any expected frequency gets to five or thereabouts.

C.R.A.P. Detector X-3

People often forget that they have matched or before–after measurements. In general, using unpaired tests on these data results in conservative tests.

11

Nonparametric Measures of Association

> Several nonparametric measures of association, equivalent to the correlation coefficient, have been devised. These include the *contingency coefficient*, the *phi coefficient*, and *Cohen's kappa coefficient*, for nominal data, and also include *Spearman's rho, Kendall's tau*, and *Kendall's W*, for ordinal data.

$You\ will\ recall$ that just about the time we had conquered the complexities of multiple group comparisons and factorial analysis of variance (ANOVA) in the section on parametric statistics, we were hauled up short by the recognition that not all questions can be addressed by throwing folks into groups. At that point, we regressed (pun) to a study of correlation and regression, methods used to measure the amount of association among two or more interval variables measured in a single sample. When we did this, we found that in addition to determining whether or not an association was statistically significant, we could also express the strength of the association by a correlation coefficient that ranged between –1 and 1.

In this chapter, we examine a number of ways to achieve the same end for nominal and ordinal data. We are seeking a coefficient that can be used on these data and that ideally will have a value of +1 when there is a perfect relationship between the two variables (which exists when one variable can be predicted exactly from knowledge of the other), –1 when there is a perfect inverse relationship, and 0 when there is no relationship between the two variables.

As usual, things aren't quite so clear-cut when you get to nonparametric measures of association. We will discuss three measures that are applicable to nominal data: the **contingency coefficient**, the **phi coefficient**, and **Cohen's kappa coefficient**. Three other measures require ordinal ranks: the

Spearman's rank correlation, Kendall's tau coefficient, and another coefficient by the prolific Dr. Kendall, the Kendall W coefficient. As usual, they all give different answers and have different strengths and weaknesses, which we'll point out as we go along.

MEASURES OF ASSOCIATION FOR NOMINAL VARIABLES

At first glance, anyone steeped in the tradition of correlation coefficients might view the idea of a measure of association for nominal variables as somewhat preposterous. After all, when you calculate a correlation coefficient, you are measuring the degree to which someone who is high or low on one variable will be high or low on another. Nominal variables are completely egalitarian and unprejudiced. None are higher or lower than any others; they are just different. But the idea of association for nominal variables is not that ridiculous. For nominal variables, the idea of association relates to frequencies in categories. Because most men have beards and relatively few women shave daily, it is natural to conclude that sex and facial hair are associated, without having to decide whether shaving is higher or lower than not shaving.

To explore the question further, let's focus on that dreaded scourge of mankind, Somaliland camel-bite fever. Fortunately, we are no longer devastated by this disease, thanks to a dedicated investigator who discovered that the serum sage level can diagnose the early stages of the disease so that treatment can be implemented. How reliable is the test? Suppose we have test results for 100 patients being treated for fever and 100 controls and that the sage test has two values, ripe and raw. The results are displayed in Table 11-1.

It certainly looks as if there is an association between a positive test result and the scourge: 80% of patients versus 30% of normals have a ripe sage. If we wanted to test whether or not the association is statistically significant (ie, different from zero) we could calculate a chi-square (χ^2), which turns out to be equal to 50.51 and which is highly significant.

Table 11-1

Comparison of Serum Sage Levels in Controls and Patients with Somaliland Camel-Bite Fever

Test Result	Patients	Controls	Totals
Ripe	80	30	110
Raw	20	70	90
Total	100	100	200

Contingency Coefficient

However, the question we address in this chapter is not whether the association is present or absent but whether there is some way to develop standard measures of the degree of association in order to compare one set of variables to another. The simplest measure is the contingency coefficient, which is based directly on the calculated χ^2. It is calculated as:

$$C = \sqrt{\frac{\chi^2}{(N + \chi^2)}}$$

where N is the sample size. In this case, the contingency coefficient is equal to:

$$C = \sqrt{\frac{50.5}{200 + 50.5}} = 0.45$$

The coefficient seems to do some of the right things; the larger χ^2 is, the closer the value will be to 1, and it has the virtue of being easy to calculate. Unfortunately, the beast has one undesirable property, namely, it doesn't go to 1 when there is a perfect relationship. In the present example, if the sage test were perfect, chi-square would equal 200 and the coefficient would equal 0.707.

Phi Coefficient

The phi coefficient is a ratio of two quantities, determined as follows. We label the four cells in a contingency table a, b, c, and d, by convention, as shown in Table 11-2.

If there is no association between test and disease, the two ratios a/b and c/d would be equal and would also be equal to the proportion of people in the sample who have the disease. So the ratio of these two numbers would be 1, and if we subtract 1 from this ratio of ratios, we end up with a number related to the degree of association between the two variables. Playing around a bit with the algebra, we have:

$$\frac{(a/b)}{(c/d)} - 1 = \frac{(ad - bc)}{bc}$$

Table 11-2
Contingency Table Depicting Ratios

	Disease Present	Disease Absent	Totals
Positive	a	b	a + b
Negative	c	d	c + d
Total	a + c	b + d	N

Actually, the phi coefficient uses a different denominator, made up of the product of the marginals:

$$\phi = \frac{ad - bc}{\sqrt{(a + b)(c + d)(a + c)(b + d)}} = \frac{80 \times 70 - 20 \times 30}{} = 0.50$$

If there is strong association, b and c equal zero, so phi becomes:

$$\phi = \frac{ad}{\sqrt{a \times d \times a \times d}} = 1$$

And if there is no association, ad = bc, and phi = 0. So it looks as if phi does the right thing at the extremes.

Cohen's Kappa Coefficient

There is one other simple measure of association that deserves a bit of mention. The upper left cell in a contingency table (positive test, disease present) and the bottom right cell (negative test, disease absent) are cells where there is agreement between test and standard. One simple way to look at association would be to ask what proportion of cases result in agreement; in this case:

$$\frac{(80 + 70)}{200} = 0.75$$

Unfortunately, this simple approach has serious problems. Certainly, the upper limit is okay. If there is perfect association, all the cases will be in these two cells. But if there is no association at all, there would be

$$\frac{(110 \times 100)}{200} = 55$$

cases in the top left and

$$\frac{(90 \times 100)}{200} = 45$$

cases in the bottom right cell. The agreement equals

$$\frac{(55 + 45)}{200} = 0.50$$

Cohen started from the notion of agreement on the diagonal cells as a measure of association but corrected for chance agreement. In our example, the actual agreement was 0.75, and chance agreement, as calculated above, was 0.5.

The formula for kappa (κ) is

$$\kappa = \frac{\text{observed agreement} - \text{chance agreement}}{1 - \text{chance agreement}}$$

So, in this example,

$$\kappa = \frac{(0.75 - 0.5)}{(1.0 - 0.50)} = 0.50$$

If there is a perfect association, observed agreement = 1 and kappa = 1. No association puts the observed agreement equal to chance agreement and kappa = 0.

These desirable properties make kappa the measure of choice for nominal data and 2 $\times$ 2 tables. But all of the coefficients have problems when the number of categories are increased and the data are ordinal. This brings us to the coefficients designed for use on ordinal data.

MEASURES OF ASSOCIATION FOR ORDINAL VARIABLES

Spearman's Rank Correlation Coefficient (Rho)

Time for another example. At last count, our colleagues in rheumatology had devised about 30 ways to tell how sick a patient with rheumatoid arthritis is, ranging from the sublime (serum this and that levels) to the ridiculous (how long it takes to stagger the 100-yard dash). Unfortunately, the relationship among all these measures is a bit underwhelming. Let's look at two old favorites: (1) joint count (JC), which, as the name implies, is a count of the number of inflamed joints, and (2) clinician rating (CR), which is a test that gives clinical judgment its due. JC is a ratio variable, but frequently, each joint is rated on a three-point scale, which makes the measure more ordinal. The CRs are on a 10-point scale. The data for eight patients are displayed in Table 11-3.

You may notice that, in good nonparametric style, we determined the ranks of each patient on JC and CR in addition to the absolute number. We could go ahead and calculate a Pearson correlation on the original data, but a quick look at the data shows that the numbers are hardly normally distributed and that they are ordinal in any case. So there is good justification to go the nonparametric route.

The basis of Spearman's correlation (denoted by R_S or rho) is the difference in ranks of each pair. If the two variables were perfectly correlated, the patient ranked highest on JC would also be highest on CR. In other words, there would be a perfect correspondence in ranks of each patient on the two variables: 1–1, 2–2, and on, down to 8–8. The difference in ranks for

Table 11-3

Comparison of Joint Count and Clinician Rating in the Assessment of Polyarthritis

Patient	Joint Count	Rank	Clinician Rating	Rank
A	85	2	9	1
B	20	6	3.5	5
C	60	4	6	3
D	25	5	1	8
E	95	1	8	2
F	70	3	5	4
G	10	8	2	7
H	15	7	3	6

each pair would all be zero. Conversely, if there were a perfect inverse relationship, the ranked pairs would look like 1–8, 2–7, 3–6,... 8–1.

Spearman, in deriving the formula that won him international acclaim, began with the formula for the product-moment correlation but proceeded to calculate the correlation for pairs of ranks rather than raw data. We won't bore you with the details, but it turns out that some simplifications emerge. In the end, the equivalent formula to the Pearson correlation for ranked data becomes the following:

$$R_S = 1 - 6 \times (\text{sum of } d^2)$$

where d is the difference in ranks on the two variables, and where N is the number of people. In our example, R_S turns out to be 0.81.

More generally, it is evident that if the data were perfectly correlated, each d would be 0, and the correlation would equal 1. If the data were inversely correlated, it turns out that the correlation is −1. So Spearman's little gem has the desirable characteristic of having appropriate upper and lower limits. But although it is derived directly from the product-moment correlation, it is only 91% as efficient as the Pearson correlation when the distributions really are normal.

Kendall's Tau

Kendall's tau is used under the same circumstances as Spearman's correlation. Of course, the approach is different. Kendall's tau has the dubious advantage that it requires no algebra, only counts. It has the disadvantage that it yields a different and lower answer than Spearman's correlation using the same data although it is preferred when there are a lot of tied ranks.

So here we go again. The data from our study have been re-arranged slightly so that the JC ranks are in ascending order.

Table 11-4
Joint Count and Clinician Rating on 8 Patients

Test	Patient							
	E	A	F	C	D	B	H	G
Joint Count	1	2	3	4	5	6	7	8
Clinical Rating	2	1	4	3	8	5	6	7

Having ordered the JC ranks, the question is, "How many of the possible pairs of CR ranks are in the right order?" A pairwise comparison is done, with +1 assigned to pairs that are in the right order, and −1 to pairs that aren't. If there were a perfect relationship, every pair would be assigned a +1, so there would be as many +1's as there were pairs.

This is how it works in this example:

2–1, 2–4, 2–3, 2–8, 2–5, 2–6, 2–7, 1–4, 1–3, 1–8, 1–5, 1–6, 1–7, 4–3,
−1, +1, +1, +1, +1, +1, +1, +1, +1, +1, +1, +1, +1, −1

4–8, 4–5, 4–6, 4–7, 3–8, 3–5, 3–6, 3–7, 8–5, 8–6, 8–7, 5–6, 5–7, 6–7,
+1, +1, +1, +1, +1, +1, +1, +1, −1, −1, −1, +1, +1, +1

The positive and negative numbers are then summed to 23 −5 = 18. This sum is divided by the maximum possible score, which is $N(N − 1)/2 = 28$ (ie, the number of pairs). So for these data, tau is equal to 18/28 = 0.64, which compares to 0.81 for the Spearman coefficient. Perhaps this is not surprising since the coefficient, like the sign test, uses only the direction and not the magnitude of the differences. Although it is conservative, it is better when there are many tied ranks. However, tau is restricted to only two groups. Perhaps that's why Dr. Kendall invented another coefficient.

Kendall's W (Coefficient of Concordance)

One problem shared by all of the coefficients discussed so far is that, like the standard Pearson correlation, they can only consider the association between two variables at a time. The occasion may arise when one might wish to determine the overall agreement among several variables. This situation often emerges in examining the agreement among multiple raters or the association among more than two variables.

Suppose a researcher wanted to obtain ratings of the interpersonal skills of a group of physical therapy students from patients, supervisors, and peers. The question now is the extent of agreement among the three ratings of each student. Using six therapists, suppose their ratings on a scale ended up ranked like this:

Table 11-5
Ranking of Six Students by Patients, Supervisors, and Peers

Student	Patient	Supervisor	Peer	Sum of Ranks
A	1	2	3	6
B	2	1	1	4
C	3	3	2	8
D	4	6	4	14
E	5	4	6	15
F	6	5	5	16

In the right-hand column, we have taken the liberty of summing the ranks for each therapist. If there were perfect agreement among the observers, then therapist A would be ranked first by everyone, and therapist F would be ranked last by all. Thus, the summed rank for A would be 1 × (number of observers)—in this case 3—and for F would be (number of therapists) × (number of observers) = 6 × 3 = 18. By contrast, if there were no association, then every summed rank would end up about the same. So one measure of the degree of association would be to determine the difference between individual rank sums and the mean rank sum. Of course, statisticians have a reflex response to square every difference they encounter, and this case is no exception. The starting point in calculating Kendall's W is to determine the summed rank for each case and the average summed rank, take the difference for each case, and add up the square of all the differences.

In our example, the average summed rank is

$$\frac{(6 + 4 + 8 + 14 + 15 + 16)}{6} = 10.5$$

So the sum of the squared deviations is

$$(6 - 10.5)^2 + (4 - 10.5)^2 + (8 - 10.5)^2 + \ldots + (16 - 10.5)^2 = 131.5$$

Now the challenge is to figure out the maximum value that this sum of squares could achieve. A little algebra (trust us) demonstrates that this is equal to

$$\frac{K^2 (N^3 - N)}{12} = \frac{(3)^2 (6^3 - 6)}{12} = \frac{1(9)(216 - 6)}{12} = 157.5$$

where K is the number of rates and N is the number of subjects.

So the coefficient of association now is simply the ratio of the actual sum of squared differences to the maximum possible (ie, 131.5/157.5 = 0.83). And that's that! By the way, application of this formula to the data used for Spearman's correlation yields a value in Table 11-3 of 0.91, versus 0.81 for R_S and 0.64 for tau.

MEASURES OF MAGNITUDE OF EFFECT

There are two indices that are used in studies that look at the effects, both good and bad, of some variable on an outcome: the **relative risk**, or **risk ratio** (RR), and the **odds ratio** (OR), or **relative odds**. The variable can be either one that's under our control, such as the patients getting a drug versus a placebo, or some factor that may increase the probability of an outcome, such as exposure to asbestos increasing the risk of mesothelioma. Let's do some real research, and see how we can use these two measures.

In a previous chapter, we introduced you to that dread disorder, photonumerophobia—the fear that our fear of numbers will come to light. We believe that this book is such a painless introduction to statistics that it can alleviate this condition in any photonumerophobic who reads it. To put this to a test, we take 200 patients, randomly give *PDQ Statistics* to half and some other book to half, and see who's phobic 6 months later. The results of this **randomized controlled trial** (RCT) are shown in Table 11-6. (See Chapter 21 for a description of an RCT.)

Obviously, something's going on. But not everyone who read the book improved (they must have just skimmed it), and some people who read the other book did in fact get better. So just how effective was *PDQ Statistics*? For those who were assigned to this book, the *risk* of not improving is a / (a + b), which is 40/100, or 0.40. At the same time, the risk of not improving after having read the other book is c / (c + d), or 80/100, or 0.80. So the relative risk (ie, the *risk* of the outcome in the group of interest *relative* to the other group) is the ratio of these, which is 0.40 / 0.80 = 0.5. In other words, people who read our book are only half as likely to fail as the poor benighted souls who were assigned the other book. Writing this out more formally yields the following:

Table 11-6
Results of Randomized Trial Comparing *PDQ Statistics* versus Another Book in Treatment of Photonumerophobia

Exposure	Outcome		Total
	Not Improved	Improved	
PDQ Stats	40 (a)	60 (b)	100 (a + b)
Other book	80 (c)	20 (d)	100 (c + d)
Total	120 (a + c)	80 (b+d)	200 (N)

$$RR = \frac{a}{a+b} \bigg/ \frac{c}{c+d} = \frac{a(c+d)}{c(a+b)}$$

(We could switch the two columns in the table and talk about the "risk" of improving—and some people actually do—but this use of the term "risk" strikes us as somewhat bizarre.)

If we were cheap (some "friends" would say cheap*er*) and didn't want to spend money giving away our books, much less someone else's, we could find 50 phobics who had bought *PDQ Statistics* and 50 who had bought that other book on their own, and we could see what happened to them. This would be called a **cohort study** (again, see Chapter 21), and we would analyze the results in the same way.

But there's even a third way to do the study. We can go through the files of the mental health clinic and find 100 *cases* (people who have been cured of photonumerophobia) and an equal number of matched *controls* (those who haven't been cured) and look back to see what book they were exposed to; for obvious reasons, this is called a **case-control study** (yet again, see Chapter 21). The results are shown in Table 11-7.

This time, we can't use the RR. The reason we can't is that we did the study by deliberately selecting 100 people who got better and 100 who did not, so we have no idea what the real ratio is between these two groups. What we can do is figure out the **odds** of having read *PDQ Statistics*, given that the person has improved (we can talk about *improvement* because we're using the word "odds" rather than "risk"), relative to the odds of improvement, given that the person hasn't read this therapeutic tome. The odds of improving with this book are 70:30 whereas they're 25:75 for the other book; so the OR is:

$$OR = \frac{a/c}{b/d} = \frac{ad}{bc}$$

which is $(70 \times 75) / (25 \times 30) = 7.0$. If we had figured out the RR, we would have found it to be only 2.58. This is a universal truth: *the OR overestimates the RR, except when the number of cases is relatively low*, say, under 5%.

Table 11-7
Results of Case-Control Study of Cured and Uncured Photonumerophobics

Exposure	Outcome Improved	Not Improved	Total
PDQ Stats	70 (a)	25 (b)	95 (a + b)
Other book	30 (c)	75 (d)	105 (c + d)
Total	100 (a + c)	100 (b + d)	200 (N)

WEIGHTED KAPPA

In a follow-up to his original paper on kappa, Cohen proposed a more general form, which could be used for ordinal data. Consider two observers using a seven-point scale to rate 100 patients. We could display all the data in a 7 × 7 matrix, with Observer 1 in the rows and Observer 2 in the columns, so that total agreement would be all the cells on the main diagonal. Now we could calculate the observed and expected proportions (the latter using the marginals).

But if I say 6 and you say 5, that's a lot closer than if I say 1 and you say 7. Cohen proposed a general form where we *weight* the degree of disagreement. Although the weights could be anything, the most rational course (for reasons which need not concern us) is to use what are called **quadratic weights**, whereby the proportions are multiplied by the square of the disagreement. If we disagree by 1, we multiply by 1. If we disagree by 2, we multiply by 4, and so on. We then calculate the sum of the weighted disagreements actually observed (q_o) and those expected by chance, based on the marginals (q_e). Then, weighted kappa (κ_w) is just:

$$\kappa_w = 1 - \frac{q_0}{q_e}$$

While not a true measure of association, weighted kappa is used universally as a measure of agreement when the data are ordinal.

That about brings us to the end of the potpourri of measures of association and agreement. Focusing on the measures applied to ordinal data, Spearman's rho coefficient is far and away the winner of the popularity poll in terms of actual usage. Kendall's W is very similar and has the advantage that it can be used as a measure of association for multiple observations. Kendall's tau is a little different and has three advantages: it is a little easier to calculate, it is better for tied ranks, and it can be used to calculate partial correlations (an area we didn't touch on). But it gives considerably lower answers in general than the other two coefficients.

C.R.A.P. DETECTORS

Example 11-1

Suppose we choose to look at interrater agreement of back mobility judgments by chiropractors. Two methods are advocated: (1) direct estimation of range of motion in degrees and (2) clinician ratings of hypermobility, normal range, and restricted range.

Question. What coefficients would you use? Any guesses as to which would be larger?

Answer. Because range of motion in degrees is ratio, Pearson's correlation would be best. However, if more than two raters are involved, Kendall's W would give a good overall picture of rater agreement. You might use kappa for clinician ratings, but these are actually crude ordinal data, so a coefficient based on ranks would be better. The loss of information in the three-point scale implies that the kappa would be lower.

C.R.A.P. Detector XI-1

If the data are reasonably interval and normal, as with many rating scales, Pearson's correlation is best.

C.R.A.P. Detector XI-2

A similar argument holds within the nonparametric domain. Measures for nominal data (such as kappa) will give low values when applied to ordinal data, in comparison to the appropriate ordinal measures.

C.R.A.P. Detector XI-3

People often use multiple raters and then calculate agreement between raters 1 and 2, 1 and 3, 7 and 8, and so on. Generally, any differences among rater pairs usually reflect statistical variation, and an overall measure of agreement such as Kendall's W is much preferred.

Advanced Nonparametric Methods

12

There are two approaches to handling designs in which the dependent variable (DV) involves frequencies in categories with more than one independent variable (IV). *Mantel-Haenszel chi-square* deals with two independent factors. *Log-linear analysis* can handle any number of IVs and multiple categorical variables, and estimates effects and interactions, analogous to factorial analysis of variance (ANOVA).

On reflection, you may realize that something is missing from the preceding two chapters. None of the methods we considered goes beyond the equivalent of one-way ANOVA or simple correlations; they all consider only two variables at a time.

Naturally, this void hasn't escaped the notice of statisticians. Several methods have been developed to deal with the relation among multiple IVs and a counted DV. The **Mantel-Haenszel chi-square** handles two categorical IVs. **Log-linear analysis** estimates frequencies in which there are multiple categorical IVs.

MANTEL-HAENSZEL CHI-SQUARE

The simplest clinical trial involves randomly assigning patients to one of two categories such as drug or placebo or such as treatment A versus treatment B. An outcome event such as death or relapse is then counted in each group, and the frequencies are compared, using a chi-square test.

One common refinement of this approach is called **prognostic stratifi-cation.** If, for example, age is likely to be associated with the outcome event (ie, old folks are more likely to die during the course of the study), then the sample is stratified to ensure that equal numbers of folks in each age group end up in the two groups. It is still legitimate simply to compare event rates in the two large groups, but it is also desirable to examine events in each age subgroup to test whether treatment effects are consistent across all ages.

A similar situation arises in studies of risk factors for disease. Having demonstrated, by assembling a series of patients who got the disease and controls who didn't, that patients are more likely to have been exposed to a particular noxious agent, we might want to show that the effect is consistent across all age and sex subgroups.

As an example, suppose we want to examine the relationship between hepatitis B and the punker practice of inserting safety pins in earlobes and noses. Because other practices in this subculture, such as using injectable drugs, might also lead to a higher rate of hepatitis, we may wish to stratify by drug use: none, moderate, and heavy use.

We assemble a few hundred punkers with hepatitis who checked into the Liverpool General, locate a comparable group of relatively healthy punkers, and inquire about safety pin and drug use. The data are arrayed in Table 12-1.

Table 12-1
Association of Hepatitis B among Drug Users and Pin Users

Drug Use	Pin Use	Hepatitis B Yes	No	Total
None	Yes	78	40	
	No	27	75	220
Moderate	Yes	92	29	
	No	19	34	174
Heavy	Yes	60	209	
	No	5	180	454
Total		281	567	848

By inspection, there certainly appears to be an association between safety pins and hepatitis B. But there is also a relation between pin use and drug use: 54% of nondrug users use pins, compared to 59% of heavy drug users who also use pins. Because both drug use and pin use are associated with hepatitis B, simply adding the subtables together to calculate an overall chi-square is going to underestimate the effect. It's a bit like the situation in analysis of covariance. Some of the variance in the event rates can be attributed to the use of drugs, so controlling for the effect of this variable will improve the likelihood of detecting a difference attributable to the primary variable of interest, safety pins.

So how do you analyze across without committing the ultimate atrocity of repeated statistical tests? Mantel and Haenszel began with the original definition of chi-square, as we did in Chapter 10. If we focus on the upper left cell in each table (labeled "a" by convention), it's easy to figure out the expected value of "a" if there were no association between pins and hepatitis. For the "no drug" group, this is just:

$$\text{Expected Value} = \frac{(a+b) \times (a+c)}{} = \frac{118 \times 105}{} = 56.3$$

The variance of this estimate is another product of marginals:

$$\text{Variance} = \frac{(a+b)(a+c)(b+d)(c+d)}{N^2(N-1)} = \frac{105 \times 115 \times 102 \times 118}{220 \times 220 \times 219} = 13.7$$

This step can be repeated for all the subtables. The final bit of subterfuge results from adding up all the a's. If there were no associations, the sum of the a's should be normally distributed with a mean equal to the sum of the expected values and a variance equal to the sum of the variances.

The reason we focus only on the "a" cells is because the difference (observed minus expected) is the same for each of the four cells, and so is the variance term in the denominator. So including all four cells just amounts to multiplying everything by four and doesn't actually change anything. So the quantity

$$\text{Chi-square} = \frac{(\text{sum of a's} - \text{sum of expected a's})^2}{\text{sum of variances}}$$

is a chi-square that can be associated with a probability in the usual way. This is the overall test of the association between safety pins and hepatitis B and turns out to equal 94.2, a highly significant association. If we had just gone ahead and calculated a chi-square based on the summary table over all levels of drug use, the result would have been 84.3. So by controlling for drug use, we have improved the sensitivity of the test.

In a sense, the Mantel-Haenszel chi-square is the nonparametric equivalent of using a covariate in analysis of covariance. It can be used to correct for bias caused by different numbers of cases in the subgroups, to improve sensitivity of the overall test as we demonstrated above, and to investigate interactions between the two factors (ie, is the effect of safety pin use different across the levels of drug use?).

However, the Mantel-Haenszel chi-square is limited to only two IVs. Two other methods are available to handle multiple IVs: logistic regression and log-linear analysis.

Before we get to these multivariable methods, there is one special application of the Mantel-Haenszel procedure that deserves further mention. A very common situation in clinical trials, particularly those in which the variable of interest is death, is that people don't wait until the last day of the study to die. This forces researchers to construct a **life table** and invoke special methods for analysis.

LIFE TABLE (OR SURVIVAL) ANALYSIS

In most of the studies described so far, the end point occurs at some fairly definite point, which is often under the control of the researcher (eg, responses to two drugs are measured a few hours or weeks after administration, demographic and clinical or performance data are gathered at entry and exit from a program, and so forth). Some studies, though, are not as neat, and the outcome appears in its own sweet time. A prime example of this would be cancer trials, where the outcome (usually death) can occur within days after the person is entered into the trial or may not happen until many years have passed. Indeed, our interest is in how long it takes to reach this end point. ("Sir, I regret to inform you that your father has reached his end point!")

However, there are at least three methodologic problems that require the use of a different form of analysis, usually called *life table analysis* or *survival curve analysis*. The first difficulty is that patients are usually enrolled into the study over a protracted period of time. In large studies, it would be unusual to have enough diabetic or cancer patients at any one point so that they can all begin the trial on the same day. Having to follow these patients over a long interval (often years) leads to the other two difficulties. During this time, we would lose track of some people because they may move, get tired of the study, or tell us to go fly a kite, and we would have no way of knowing what happens to them. Furthermore, the funding agency may remind us that all good things, including our study, must come to an end.

So at the end of the study, rather than just the one neat end point we anticipated, our subjects have three possible outcomes: deceased (or in relapse, depending on the nature of the trial), lost to follow-up after varying periods of time, and still alive (or well) after varying periods. Complicating the issue a bit more, the "varying periods" can be the result of two different causes: (1) the dropouts can any time the patient moves or gets fed up and (2) because the patients are enrolled over the course of the study, they are at risk for different periods at the point when we stop the study.

These different possibilities are shown in Figure 12-1, where "W" indicates withdrawal and "X" means the subject died. Subjects 1, 4, 9, and 10 died during the trial; subjects 3, 6, and 7 withdrew; and subjects 2, 5, and 8 were still alive when the study ended in year 5. (The data from these last three people are referred to as "censored." This simply means that the study ended before they did, and it casts no aspersions on their moral virtues.) The question we now have to answer is, "How long do patients survive after they begin treatment?" If we base our conclusions only on the subjects for whom we have complete data, then the answer would be the mean of 30 months (subject 1), 10 months (subject 4), 14 months (subject 9), and 16 months (subject 10), or just under 1 1/2 years. This approach is unsatisfying for two reasons. First, we've discarded much of our data, and we haven't taken into account that the surviving subjects are indeed still around and kicking when we had to end the study. Second, what do we do with the withdrawals? Obviously, we can't determine length of survival from their data, but they did provide useful information before they withdrew.

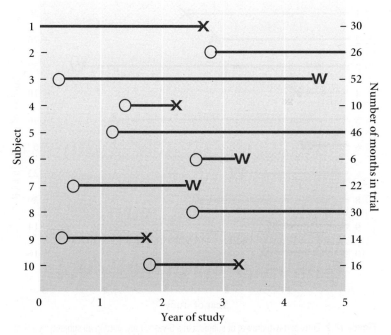

Figure 12-1 Entry and withdrawal of subjects in a 5-year study.

We can get around some of these problems in a way dear to a researcher's heart: if we don't like the answer, let's change the question. What we can look at is the proportion of people who were still alive at the end of 1 year; the proportion alive at the end of 2 years if they were in the study at the end of 1 year, and so on. To make our job easier, let's redraw Figure 12-1 so that it looks as if everyone started at the same time. This yields Figure 12-2, where "W" and "X" have the same meaning as before, and where "A" indicates that the person was alive when the study ended.

From this we can easily make a life table showing the number of people in the study at the start of each year, how many withdrew during that year, and how many died (Table 12-2). Note that the people who were censored (subjects 2, 5, and 8) are counted as withdrawals.

So far, so good. But how many patients died during the first year of the trial? We know for a fact that one did (subject 4), but what do we do with subject 6? He withdrew some time during the year—we're not sure exactly when—but we don't know what happened to him. Here, we make an assumption that the person withdrew halfway through the interval—in this case, 1 year. Actually, this is less of a leap of faith than it seems. If the trial is

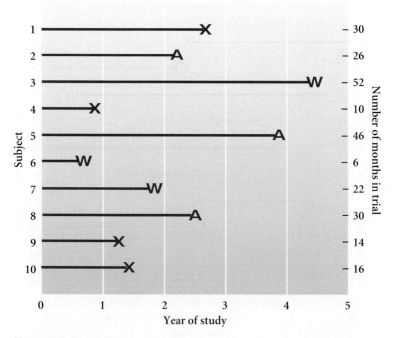

Figure 12-2 Entry and withdrawal of subjects in a 5-year study, putting all subjects at a common starting point.

Table 12-2
Life Table for the E. Ternal Longevity Study

Years in Study	Number of Patients at Risk	Number of Deaths in Year	Withdrawals during Year
0–1	10	1	1
1–2	8	2	1
2–3	5	1	2
3–4	2	0	1
4–5	1	0	1

large enough and if withdrawals occur at random, then this would simply be the mean time that these subjects are at risk.

During the first year, then, 9.5 people were at risk of dying—9 people for 1 year and 1 person for one-half year—of whom 1 actually died. So the risk of dying during the first year is 1/9.5, or 0.1053. Conversely, the probability of surviving is $1 - 0.1053$, or 0.8947. Similarly, during year 2, 7.5 people were at risk, of whom 2 died; so the probability of surviving the second year, *if you were around when the year began*, is 0.7333. The chances of surviving the entire 2-year span is the probability of making it through the first year (0.8947) times the probability of living through the interval between years 1 and 2 (0.7333), or 0.6561.

Five people entered the third year of the trial, but two withdrew. Crediting each as being at risk for half a year, we have one death in four person-years, for a probability of surviving of 0.75. Thus, the chances of surviving all 3 years is 0.6561×0.75, or 0.4921. In our admittedly sparse trial, no deaths occurred during the last 2 years, so the probabilities don't change. If we now plot the cumulative probabilities for each year, as shown in Figure 12-3, we'll have our survival curve.

Although we can get much useful information from this type of survival analysis, its real glory comes when we *compare* a number of treatments, or a treatment versus a control group, and so on. We start out exactly the same way, deriving a survival curve for each condition. Our questions now are (1) at any given point in the trial, is one arm doing better than the other? and (2) at the end of the trial, are there better overall results from one condition as compared with the other(s)? Oncologists often phrase the question the first way, such as, "Do the 5-year survival rates for breast cancer differ depending on whether or not the woman receives radiation therapy following lumpectomy?" The advantages of this approach are that it is easy to calculate and the answer is readily understood. However, the down side is that it ignores all of the information about what happens up to and after 5

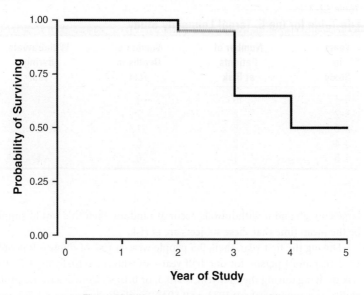

Figure 12-3 Survival curve for data in Table 12-2.

years. A more sophisticated approach uses a variation of the Mantel-Haenszel chi-square, which we've just discussed, and incorporates all of the data. Its calculation is a bit more complex than we'd like to get into, but statistical masochists can look at the grown-up version of this book if they want all the gory details.[1]

What we have just described is usually referred to as the **actuarial method** for survival analysis, in which the status of the subjects is looked at after a fixed period of time (each month, or every 6 months, or every year, depending on the length of follow-up and how frequently the end points occur). In some trials, though, we may have the actual date that a person "end-pointed" (a much nicer term than "kicked the bucket"). Here, we can use a slight modification of the technique, called the **Kaplan-Meier (K-M) approach**. The major difference between it and the actuarial method is that rather than calculating the probability of survival only at the fixed intervals, the K-M analysis calculates it only when an end point occurs. So it's possible that there may be 6 months between the first and second analyses but only 2 days between the second and third. The K-M method is usually more efficient than the actuarial method when there are fewer than 50 subjects, but the differences between the results are quite minor for the most part.

[1]Norman GR, Streiner DL. *Biostatistics: the bare essentials.* (2nd ed.). Toronto: BC Decker; 2000.

ADJUSTING FOR COVARIATES

When we looked at various ANOVA models, we mentioned that it is often necessary and worthwhile to adjust for baseline differences among the groups, using analysis of covariance (ANCOVA). A similar situation exists with survival analysis. Despite our best efforts in randomizing subjects to the various conditions, group differences that could conceivably affect the outcomes may still exist at baseline. Not surprisingly, a comparable technique exists for survival analysis, or to be more accurate, a family of techniques exists. If the covariate is dichotomous (eg, gender or the presence/absence of another condition), we can split the groups on the basis of that variable and use (yet again) the Mantel-Haenszel test. If the variable is continuous (eg, age or an illness severity score), we can use something called **Cox's Proportional Hazards Model**. As before, we won't get into the calculations (since no rational human would do them by hand) but rather refer you to a (ie, our) more advanced book.

ASSUMPTIONS

No matter which form of survival is used, four assumptions must be met. First, each person must have an identifiable starting point; that is, all the subjects have to enter the trial at the same time in the course of their illness, such as at the start of therapy or once a tumor reaches a certain size. Using diagnosis as an entry time can be problematic because people may have had the disorder for varying lengths of time before seeing their physicians or before the doctor recognized what was going on. Second, a clearly defined and uniform end point is required. This isn't much of a problem when the final state is the final resting place, but it can be a problem if the end point is the recurrence of symptoms or the reappearance of a growth, for the same reasons as with entry criteria. Third, the reasons that people drop out of the study cannot be related to the outcome. If it is (ie, the person didn't show for the follow-up visit because he has fled this vale of tears), then we could seriously overestimate the chances of survival. Fourth, we assume that diagnostic and treatment practices don't change over the life of the study and that a person's chances of being diagnosed and successfully (or unsuccessfully) treated are the same, whether the subject was the first one enrolled or the last. Otherwise, any changes we see may be due to these **secular changes** rather than the intervention.

LOG-LINEAR ANALYSIS

Unlike logistic regression, log-linear analysis is designed to analyze only categorical variables. Furthermore, it does not distinguish between IVs and DVs; alive/dead is just one more category like over 50/under 50 or men/women. Let's use a relatively simple three-factor case, the drug use/

hepatitis problem that began this chapter. You may wish to have another look at Table 12-1 to refresh your memory.

The basis of the log-linear analysis is a thing called an **effect**. To see how the idea comes about, let's examine what the data would look like if there was no association at all among all the factors. The frequency in each cell would be predicted exactly by the product of the marginals, using the same approach that was first introduced in the chi-square test.

Bringing in a little algebra, let U_1 be the proportion of nonusers in the sample:

$$U_1 = \frac{(78 + 40 + 27 + 75)}{848} = 0.259$$

Similarly, we can calculate the proportion of moderate (U_2) and heavy (U_3) users. Using different marginals, we can also calculate the expected proportions for the safety pin use (S_1 and S_2) and for hepatitis B (H_1 and H_2). Then the expected value of each cell, under the hypothesis of no association, is the total sample size, 848, times the product of the appropriate proportions. So, for example, the expected frequency in the moderate use/safety pin/hepatitis cell is:

$$\text{Expected frequency} = 848 \times (U_2 \times S_1 \times H_1) = 34.5$$

The alternative to no association in this problem is *some* association, but there are several possible associations that can be considered, namely, between hepatitis and pin use (call it HS), between hepatitis and drug use (HU), between drug use and pin use (US), or among all three (HUS). In the most extreme case, all may be important, so the frequency in a cell will be predicted from all of the two-way and three-way proportions:

$$F_{211} = N \times U_2 \times S_1 \times H_1 \times US_{21} \times UH_{21} \times HS_{11} \times HUS_{121}$$

The situation is analogous to factorial ANOVA, in which there can be main effects, two-way, three-way, and four-way interactions, with separate tests of significance for each one.

Now comes the magic act. Up until now, numbers aren't logarithmic, and they aren't linear. However, it turns out that the logarithm of a product of terms is just the sum of the logs of the individual terms. If we call the logs of our original terms by a different name, so that $\log U_1 = u_1$, then the following results:

$$\log(F_{211}) = n + u_2 + s_1 + h_1 + us_{21} + uh_{21} + hs_{11} + hus_{121}$$

So by taking the log, we have created a linear model. This, of course, causes great delight among statisticians, who can go ahead and calculate coefficients with gay abandon. However, the equation we developed is only one model. We began with the "no-association" model, which looks like the following:

$$\log(F_{211}) = n + u_2 + s_1 + h_1$$

Actually, there is a family of models, depending on which associations (or effects) are significant. The usual approach is to proceed in a hierarchical fashion, starting with no association, until an adequate fit is achieved. Fit is measured, as with logistic regression, by an overall goodness-of-fit chi-square and chi-squares on the individual coefficients. If the no-association model fits the data, there's no reason to proceed. But if it doesn't, two-way interaction effects are introduced one at a time, then in combination, until an adequate fit is obtained and the addition of additional effects does not significantly improve the fit.

The alternative strategy is to start with the full-blown model to get a sense of which coefficients are significant and then test reduced models based on this information. The computer is indifferent to the strategy, so both approaches should lead to the same point.

We have pretty well exhausted the possibilities for handling a single categorical DV. Logistic regression (Chapter 8) and log-linear analysis handle multiple IVs. With log-linear, everything must be dichotomous; with logistic, there are no restrictions. Survival analysis handles the case where the outcome may occur at varying times. As with many complex approaches, these methods can be subject to abuse, as the following example illustrates.

C.R.A.P. DETECTOR

Example 12-1

A multicenter trial was conducted, comparing surgical and medical management of angina. Surgical treatment entailed the use of bypass grafts, and had an operative mortality of 5%. Five hundred patients were enrolled in each group and were observed for an average of 1.5 years. At the end, there were 35 deaths in the surgical group and 20 deaths in the medical group. The difference was significant (chi-square = 4.33, $p = 0.05$).

Question. Would you choose medical therapy?

Answer. No way. If you exclude perioperative mortality, there were only 10 deaths in the surgical treatment group versus 20 in the medically treated group. Patients were followed-up for only 1.5 years; a longer follow-up period probably would have favored surgical intervention.

C.R.A.P. Detector XII-1

More errors are committed through failure to use life table analysis than by using it. You should have a good idea of when the deaths occurred, and this is best achieved with a life table.

Part Four

Multivariate Statistics

13

Introduction to Multivariate Statistics

Around the turn of the century, any charlatan could sell a healing device to a gullible customer simply by saying that it was based on the principles of electricity or magnetism. These fields were in their infancy, and what they did seemed almost magical or miraculous, so that it was difficult for the general public to differentiate between valid and fanciful claims. Being much wiser and more sophisticated now, we would not be taken in by such a sales pitch or fooled by such a fallacious appeal to science. Or would we?

It seems that today's equivalent of electricity is multivariate statistics, which has the aura of science around it and is poorly understood by the uninitiated. It would be unusual to find an article entitled, "A *t* test of . . ." or "A nonparametric analysis of . . .," but we do see many articles that begin with, "A multivariate analysis of . . .," as though what follows must be truth and beauty. This isn't to say that people who use multivariate statistics are charlatans but rather that if multivariate statistics are used, then we often suspend our critical judgment and assume that the conclusions are not only valid but perhaps even more valid than if univariate statistics had been used.

Multivariate statistics do have some advantages and are clearly indicated in some circumstances, but unfortunately, they also have disadvantages. George Bernard Shaw, in his marvelous play *The Doctor's Dilemma*, had the crusty old physician say, "Chloroform has done a lot of mischief. It's enabled every fool to be a surgeon." In the same way, SPSS and SAS (two of the most popular sets of "canned" programs) have allowed everybody to be a statistician, whether or not they understand what they are doing, and we have been inundated with highly complex analyses of completely inappropriate data. In this section, we explore what multivariate statistics are, what their results mean, and when they should or should not be used.

WHAT DO WE MEAN BY "MULTIVARIATE?"

"Multivariate" means just what it sounds like it means: many variables. In statistical jargon, it has an even narrower meaning: many dependent variables (DVs). (Like the fabled Hungarian nobleman who could only count to three, statisticians call anything more than one, many.) Let's say you want to see if salt-free diets are as effective in reducing hypertension in thin people as in obese individuals. One study could be structured with two groups of men, one of men at least 25% over their ideal body weight and one of men at or below ideal weight. Half of each group would be put on a salt-free diet, and the other half would remain on their regular diets. You will measure their diastolic blood pressure 1 month later. This would not be considered a multivariate design since there is only one dependent measure, diastolic blood pressure (DBP). The other two variables, weight and diet, are independent variables (IVs), so you could stick with a univariate test such as an analysis of variance (ANOVA).

But if you want to look at both DBP and, say, low-density lipoprotein (LDL) cholesterol, you've just graduated to the big time and will have to use one of the multivariate tests. You may wonder why there is this sudden conceptual leap when all you are doing is measuring a second DV. Why not simply do two or three separate ANOVAs?

There are two major reasons, both having to do with the fact that any time you measure two or more variables for the same person, those variables are correlated to some degree. Staying with the present example, if you know a person's DBP is 80, you could probably guess his cholesterol level. You won't know the exact level, but you'd be more accurate than if you didn't know his DBP. Testing each variable separately with univariate statistics is a bit unfair. If a significant difference were found between the groups for diastolic pressure, then you would expect to see a difference for LDL cholesterol level, simply because the two are correlated. The two analyses are not independent.

The second reason is almost the obverse of the first. Just as the interaction among IVs in a factorial ANOVA provides new information that cannot be found by examining each variable separately, the simultaneous observation of two or more DVs provides more information than a series of separate univariate analyses.

Just to give some life to these concepts, consider the (fictitious) data in Table 13-1. We have two groups, treatment and control, and the two DVs, DBP and LDL cholesterol. If we did a *t* test on DBP, we'd find a value of 1.55 with 48 degrees of freedom, which is far from being statistically significant. For LDL, the value of *t* would be 1.90, again not significant. We could plot the distributions of the two variables for the groups, as we've done in Figures 13-1 and 13-2, which reinforce our impression that the groups are

Table 13-1

Comparison of Blood Pressure and Serum Cholesterol between Treatment and Control Groups

	Treatment Group	Control Group
Diastolic Blood Pressure mm Hg		
Mean	87	95
Standard deviation	15	21
LDL Cholesterol mmol/L		
Mean	2.53	2.09
Standard deviation	0.84	0.79
Sample Size	25	25

fairly similar. If we really want to milk the data for all they're worth, we could calculate a point-biserial correlation between each variable and group membership (1 if treatment group, 2 if control group). Not surprisingly, we won't find much, just a correlation of -0.12 for DBP and 0.10 for LDL, which don't differ significantly from zero. So if we were limited to univariate statistics, we would have to unpack our bags at this point since we wouldn't be going to the next Nobel Prize ceremony in Stockholm. But if we use multivariate statistics, we'd get a highly significant result. In the next few chapters, we'll see why the results from the multivariate and the univariate analyses yield such different findings.

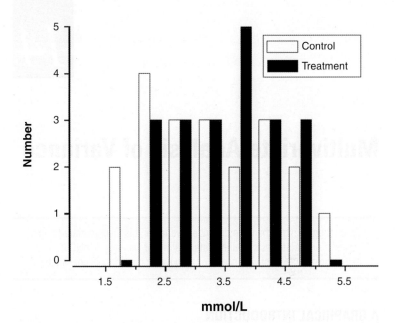

Figure 13-1 Distribution of the low-density lipoprotein (LDL) scores for the treatment and control groups.

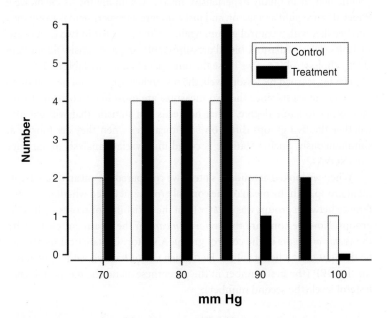

Figure 13-2 Distribution of the diastolic blood pressure (DBP) scores for the treatment and control groups.

14

Multivariate Analysis of Variance

When there is more than one dependent variable, it is inappropriate to do a series of univariate tests. Multivariate analysis of variance (MANOVA) is an extension of analysis of variance, used with two or more dependent variables.

A GRAPHICAL INTRODUCTION

Let's return to the example of seeing if salt reduction has any therapeutic benefit in mildly hypertensive males. To simplify the problem, we'll forget about weight as a factor, and just compare an experimental group on a salt-free diet with a control group. Again, we're interested in two dependent variables (DVs)—diastolic blood pressure (DBP) and low-density lipoprotein (LDL) cholesterol—and we'll use the same data that are in Table13-1.

Having learned his lessons well, the researcher realizes that he cannot do two separate *t* tests since the two measures are most likely correlated with each other to some degree. What he needs is a statistic that will tell him whether the two groups differ on *both* measures when they are looked at simultaneously. Such a statistic is called multivariate analysis of variance (MANOVA).

When we looked at Student's *t* test, we compared the mean of the treatment group with the mean of the control group and tested whether this difference between groups was greater than the variability of scores within the groups. Now we compare the *vector of means* in the treatment group with the *vector of means* in the control group. A **vector**, in statistical terms, can be thought of as a list of values. Here, each vector has two values: the mean for the DBP (the first number in the parentheses) and the mean LDL cholesterol level (the second number):

$$x_t = (87, 2.53) \qquad x_c = (95, 2.09)$$

130

We are not limited to two means per group; MANOVA can handle any number of DVs. If the researcher had also measured the serum aldosterone level, then he could still use MANOVA, and the vector for each group would then consist of three values.

In Figure 14-1, we have plotted what the data might look like, with cholesterol on one axis and DBP on the other. The center of each ellipse is shown as C_t for the treatment group and C_c for the control group. Actually, C_t is plotted at the point where the mean values of cholesterol and DBP intersect for the control group, and C_c is plotted similarly. Statisticians, of course, like obscure words, and so these points are called the **centroids** of the groups.

The distance between the two means is obvious; just connect the two centroids, and measure the length of the line. This can also be done algebraically as Euclid demonstrated 2,000 years ago. The algebra naturally covers more than two variables, even if graph paper doesn't; it's just a matter of connecting two points in 3-, 4-, or n-dimensional space.

Now let's get back to our original question: Do these two points (or centroids, or vectors of means) differ from each other? The answer is, we still don't know. As in the case of Student's t test, we have to know a bit more about the data. In the univariate test, this information consists of the **variance** or **standard deviation** of the data. In the multivariate case, we need this too, plus one other bit of information, the correlation between (or among) the variables.

Armed with the wisdom of the variability of scores gleaned from the previous chapters, the reasons for including the variance are self-evident to you. But, you may wonder why we've brought in the correlation coefficient, almost as if from left field.

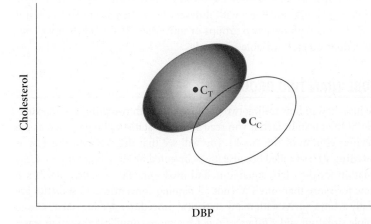

Figure 14-1 Diastolic blood pressure (DBP) and cholesterol in treatment and control groups

Let's go back to Figure 14-1. The size and shape of the ellipse tell us that the two variables are correlated positively with one another; that is, a high value on DBP is usually associated with a high value for cholesterol, and vice versa. We can take one of the groups—say, the treatment group—as the standard and look at where the centroid for the other group falls. Notice that the mean value for DBP is *higher* in the control group than in the treatment group but that the mean value for cholesterol is *lower*; that is, the relationship between the two centroids is opposite to that of the variables as a whole—a higher mean on one variable is paired with a lower mean on the other. That would make this finding unusual, at least on an intuitive basis. So the correlation coefficient tells us that the two variables should be *positively* correlated, and the negative correlation between the two reflects a deviation from the overall pattern.

If the two variables were *negatively* correlated, on the other hand, we wouldn't make too much of the relationship between the centroids; it simply goes along with what the data look like as a whole.

At this point, let's assume that we've found a significant F ratio. What does all this tell us? It means that the *centroids* of the two groups are significantly different from each other. But, there are three ways in which the groups can differ: (1) they can be significantly different on variable 1 but not on variable 2, (2) they can differ on the second variable but not on the first, and (3) both variables may be significantly different. If there were three variables, then there would be seven possible ways the groups could differ; four variables would lead to 15 different ways, and so on. This test does not tell us *which* of these possibilities is actually the case, simply that *one* of them resulted in a significant F ratio. This is analogous to the omnibus F ratios we encountered with just plain analysis of variance (ANOVA); at least two of the groups differ, but we don't know which two. With MANOVA, we have to follow a significant F test with different tests, such as Student's t test if we're dealing with only two groups or univariate ANOVAs when we have more, done on each variable separately.

MORE THAN TWO GROUPS

We just showed how testing two or more DVs with two groups is an extension of the t test. In fact, if you read some old statistics books (such as the previous edition of this book), you will see that they refer to this test as **Hotelling's T²**, so called because it was invented by Hotelling, who took the equation for the t test, squared it, and used some fancy matrix algebra to allow for more than one DV (not all naming conventions in statistics are totally arbitrary). As with many statistical procedures, having one test for a simple situation and a different one for a more complicated version was a result of having to do things by hand and being on the lookout for shortcuts. Now that computers do the work for us, the distinctions don't matter, and we won't find anything called "Hotelling's T²" in any of the statistical packages. (We *will* find something called "Hotelling's trace," but that's something else entirely.)

However, having more than two groups does change how we conceptualize what we're doing. So instead of using the *t* test as a model, we have to use ANOVA and expand it to handle the situation. In ANOVA, we use an *F* ratio to determine if the groups are significantly different from each other, and the formula for this test is:

$$F = \frac{\text{mean square (treatments)}}{\text{mean square (error)}}$$

That is, we are testing whether there is greater variability between the groups (ie, the "treatments" effect) than within the groups (ie, the "error").

In the case of MANOVA, though, we do not have just one term for the treatments effect and one for the error. Rather, we have a number of treatment effects and a number of error terms. This is because in an ANOVA, each group mean could be represented by a single number whereas in a MANOVA, each group has a **vector of means**, one mean for each variable. So when we examine how much each group differs from the "mean" of all the groups combined, we are really comparing the centroid of each group to the grand centroid. Similarly, the within-group variability has to be computed for each for the DVs.

Again we calculate a ratio, but in this case, we have to divide one series of scores by another group of scores. The techniques for doing this are referred to as matrix algebra and are far beyond the scope of this book. Fortunately, though, there are many computer programs that can do this scut work for us.

However, there are two points that make our life somewhat difficult. First, we have gotten used to the idea that the larger the result of a statistical test, the more significant the findings. For some reason that surpasseth human understanding, this has been reversed in the case of MANOVA. Instead of calculating the treatment mean square divided by the error mean square, MANOVA computes the equivalent of the error term divided by the treatment term. Hence, the *smaller* this value is, the more significant the results.

The second problem, which is common to many multivariate procedures, is that we are blessed (or cursed, depending on your viewpoint) with a multitude of different ways to accomplish the same end. In MANOVA, there are many test statistics used to determine whether or not the results are significant. The most widely used method is called **Wilks' lambda**, but there are many other procedures that can be used. Arguments about which is the best one to use make the debates among the medieval Scholastics look tame and restrained. Each method has its believers, and each has its detractors. In most instances, the statistics yield equivalent results. However, if the data are only marginally significant, it's possible that one of the test statistics would say one thing and that the other tests would say the opposite; which one to believe then almost becomes a toss-up. As with Hotelling's T^2 test, a significant finding tells us only that a difference exists *somewhere* in the data, but it doesn't tell us where. For this, we use a simpler ANOVA on each variable.

Because MANOVA is simply an extension of ANOVA, we would expect that there would be a multivariate version of analysis of covariance (ANCOVA). Not surprisingly, there is one; equally unsurprisingly, it's called **multivariate analysis of covariance** (**MANCOVA**). In an analogous way, there isn't just one MANCOVA, but a family of them (eg, 2 × 2 factorial, repeated measures), each one corresponding to a univariate ANCOVA.

C.R.A.P. DETECTORS

Example 14-1

Our intrepid psoriasis researcher feels that patients who keep kosher may respond differently to clam juice than other people, and so he divides each group, based on this variable.

Question 1. What statistical procedure should he use to see if this factor affects the extent of lesion?

Answer. He would still use a univariate test, such as the *t* test. Kosher versus traif (ie, nonkosher) is an IV, so there is still only one DV, namely, lesion extent.

C.R.A.P. Detector XIV-1

Multivariate procedures are used only when there are multiple *dependent* variables, not independent ones.

Question 2. What would happen if he ran a Hotelling's T^2 test or MANOVA on the data?

Answer. Although the test statistic will be different (a Wilks' lambda or an *F* test as opposed to a *t* test), the conclusions will be the same since T^2 is a special case of MANOVA (using only two groups) and since *t* is a special case of T^2 (only one DV).

C.R.A.P. Detector XIV-2

Beware the unneeded multivariate test! It may look more impressive, but if there's only one DV, then the authors are going in for a bit of statistical overkill.

Question 3. Assume the researcher found a significant difference between kosher versus traif. Does this mean that this factor plays a role?

Answer. Not necessarily. In all multivariate procedures, the rule of thumb is that there should be at least 10 subjects per variable. With a smaller subject-to-variable ratio, any result, significant or not, is likely to be unreliable and probably wouldn't be found if the study was replicated.

C.R.A.P. Detector XIV-3

Don't regard too seriously any study that used fewer than 10 subjects for each variable.

15

Discriminant Function Analysis

When there are many dependent variables, significant differences among the groups can be due to the effect of just one variable, some of the variables, or all of them. *Discriminant function analysis* indicates which variables are most important in accounting for the differences.

$Discriminant\ function\ analysis$ (DFA) is used when we have two or more groups and when each subject is measured on at least two dependent measures. If the groups are different, we would want to know (1) on which variables they differ and (2) whether they differ more on some variables than on others. The mathematics of the technique derives a *function (ie, an equation) that best discriminates between the groups*; hence the name "discriminant function analysis." The equation is simply the first variable multiplied by a "weight," plus the second variable multiplied by its "weight," and so on for all of the variables, like this:

$$w_1V_1 + w_2V_2 + \ldots + w_pV_p$$

where the *w*'s are the weights and the *V*'s are the variables, for all of the "p" variables. This is like a regression equation, except that we are predicting group membership rather than a particular value of a dependent variable (DV).

One of the best ways to conceptualize what DFA does is to visualize it. We can begin with a relatively simple example of only two groups with two DVs. Let's imagine that a researcher wants to see why some postmyocardial infarction patients drop out of an exercise program. She divides her subjects into two groups, compliers and noncompliers, and measures two variables on each person: (1) forced expiratory volume (FEV_1), a measure of respiratory function, and (2) an index of "health belief." In the last chapter, we showed how we can summarize the results for the two groups by drawing scatterplots. We'll do the same thing again, as is shown in Figure 15-1. This time, the two axes are for the variables FEV$_1$ and health belief, and the two ellipses represent the two groups, compliers (C) and noncompliers (N).

We begin by drawing a line that would best separate these two groups from each other. This is very simple to do by hand: draw a straight line through the two points where the ellipses cross each other, and continue the line a little bit past the point where it crosses one of the axes. This is Line I in Figure 15-2.

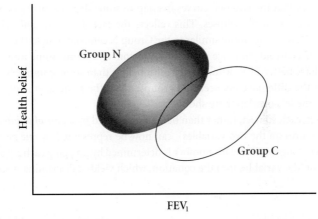

Figure 15-1 Health belief and forced expiratory volume (FEV$_1$) scores for the noncomplier (N) group and complier (C) group.

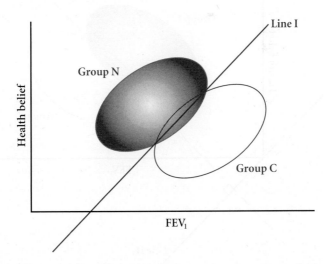

Figure 15-2 Line (Line I) that best separates noncomplier (N) and complier (C) groups on health belief and FEV$_1$.

Although the two groups fall to either side of this line, it is not the discriminant function. We now draw another line, perpendicular to the first and passing through the origin; in Figure 15-3, this is Line II. As we'll see in a short while, *this* is the discriminant function line. What we can now do is project each point in the ellipses onto Line II. This will result in two bell curves, one for each ellipse. The maximum point of the bell curve falls exactly under the centroid since this is where most of the points cluster. The farther away we get from the centroid, the fewer points there are, so the bell curve tapers off at the ends, as demonstrated in Figure 15-4.

Notice that the two bell curves overlap to some degree, corresponding to the overlap in the ellipses. This reflects the fact that some subjects in Group C have scores more similar to the Group N centroid than to their own Group C centroid, and vice versa. In more concrete terms, some noncompliers have better FEV_1 values and health beliefs than some compliers. The greater the difference between the groups, given the same degree of variability, the less overlap there should be.

First, each subject, rather than being represented by a *pair of points* (his or her scores on the two variables), can now be represented by *one point*, a number along this line. This number is determined by plugging each person's scores on the variables into the equation, which yields a discriminant score.

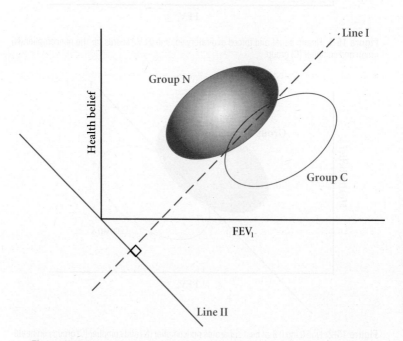

Figure 15-3 Discriminant function between complier (C) and noncomplier (N) groups.

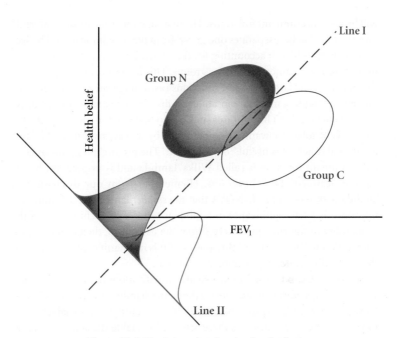

Figure 15-4 Discriminant function showing distributions.

Now for each individual subject, we can see whether his or her scores are more similar to the centroid of the compliance group or the noncompliance group. The point at which the two curves cross, under Line I, minimizes the overlap and results in the smallest number of cases being misclassified.

Let's spend a few minutes discussing the equation itself. As we said before, it includes all of the variables, and each variable is multiplied by a different weight. This should sound familiar to you since it's the same idea we discussed in relation to a regression equation. If the variables are standardized (ie, all variables have been transformed to have the same mean—zero—and the same standard deviation—one), then the larger the absolute value of the weight, the more that variable contributes to discriminating between groups. Weights close to zero indicate variables that don't add much to the discriminating power of the equation. Thus, running a DFA after a significant T^2 or multivariate analysis of variance (MANOVA) can tell us which variable the groups differ on by examining the discriminant weights, which is an alternate way of doing a post hoc test following MANOVA.

What if there are more than two groups? Except in highly unusual cases, one discriminant function won't be sufficient to discriminate among three or more groups. In fact, by the mathematics of DFA, if there are *k* groups, there will be $k - 1$ discriminant functions. The first function is the most "powerful" one, the one that best separates one group from the remaining ones. The second function is best in accounting for the remaining variance and may help in discriminating among the other groups. This pattern continues on down the line, with the last or last few functions (assuming four or more groups) possibly not adding much to our ability to discriminate among the groups.

Statisticians don't like phrases such as "doesn't add too much." Being literal sorts of folks, we want a number whereby we can say either, "Yes, this additional function is useful," or "Forget it." The test for the significance of a discriminant function is called **Wilks' lambda** and is printed out by the various "canned" DFA programs. (Remember from our discussion of lambda with respect to MANOVA that the *smaller* lambda is, the more significant it is.) The significance of lambda is tested with a chi-square; if the probability of the chi-square is less than the usual 0.05, then that function contributes to the discriminating power; if it is not significant, it (and all of the succeeding functions) can be disregarded.

Also, DFA can be used (and usually is) with more than two variables. Graphing it gets difficult, but the mathematics handles it with relative ease. However, there are two problems in adding more groups and variables. First, in general, the more variables there are, the less stable the solution is; that is, upon replication, the variables that appeared to be powerful discriminators the first time may not be so at later times. This should sound familiar since the same thing was discussed in regard to regression analysis. The second problem is that the more functions there are, the more difficult the interpretation becomes. One function is easy, two you can handle, but trying to understand three or more significant discriminant functions can be likened to deciphering the Rosetta stone without knowing any Greek. So, as the Bauhaus has taught us (and like many things in life), less is more.

In reading articles in which DFA was used, you'll probably run across the term "stepwise," as in "a stepwise solution was used." Just as in regression analysis, a stepwise solution considers variables one at a time. The equation first considers the variable that best discriminates among the groups. Then, a second variable is added, the one that most improves the discriminating ability of the equation. This process of adding one variable at a time is continued until one of two things happens: either all of the variables are entered into the equation or adding the remaining variables doesn't appreciably (read "statistically significantly") improve the power of the equation in discriminating among the groups.

The advantages and disadvantages of this procedure as discussed here are similar to those when it's used in regression analysis. On the positive side, it allows you to pick a smaller subset from a large number of variables with almost equal discriminating ability, and it ranks the variables in order of their importance. This can be very useful when it's necessary to cut down the number of variables to improve the ratio of subjects to variables, explain group differences most parsimoniously, or replicate the study with a smaller number of tests.

The primary disadvantage is an interpretive one. If two of the variables are correlated, then one may end up in the function but the other may not. The reason for this is that, as with stepwise regression, *a variable is entered if it improves the discrimination over and above any effect of the previously entered variables.* So if forced vital capacity (FVC) is highly correlated with FEV_1 and if FEV_1 has already been entered, then FVC may not give us any additional information and won't be part of the final equation. This feature is terrific if we want to select a smaller set of variables for some purpose, but it can lead us down the garden path if we conclude from this that the groups don't differ in terms of FVC. They *do* differ, but FVC doesn't explain any more of the differences than we already know about from their differences on FEV_1.

Unfortunately, there is yet another aspect to DFA: **classification analysis**. Classification analysis is a separate statistical technique that exists independently from DFA, but the two techniques are most frequently encountered together, so we'll treat them together. Recall that we can use DFA in a number of ways: to indicate on which variables two or more groups differ; to choose a subset of variables that do as good a job as the original, larger set; and to classify a given subject into a group. We'll look for a moment at the use of DFA for classification.

If we go back to Figure 15-4, each subject's scores can be plugged into the discriminant function and reduced to a single point on Line II. Then, if he or she falls on one side of the cutoff (Line I), that person can be predicted to be in the compliant group, and if on the other side, in the noncompliant group.

This type of analysis can be used in a number of ways. Perhaps the most useful although least used way is to derive a series of equations on one set of groups and then use those functions to predict where a new subject falls. The way classification analysis is *mostly* used is to check on the "goodness" of the discriminant functions. Here, the same people are used to generate the equations, and they are then "classified" by plugging their original scores back into the functions. If subject 1 was originally from group A and the equations place him closer to the A centroid, then we've got a "hit." However, if the equations say he is more similar to group B's centroid, then we have a "miss." So, for all subjects, we have two indices of group membership: the *actual* group the person is from and the group *predicted* on the basis of the equations. From this, we can construct a two-way table, with the rows being the actual group and the columns being the predicted one. Let's make up a simple example, in which group A has 100 subjects and group B has 50. The results are shown in Table 15-1.

As we can see, 75 of the subjects in group A are correctly placed using the equation, and 30 of the 50 group B subjects have been put in the right

Table 15-1
Two-Way Table to Demonstrate Accuracy of Classification

Actual Group	Predicted Group		Total
	A	B	
A	75	25	100
B	20	30	50
Total	95	55	150

group. Overall, 70% of the subjects have been correctly classified by the discriminant function. Often, a chi-square is calculated on this table to see if these results differ from a chance finding.

Moreover, most of the packaged computer programs for DFA can also tell us how confidently we can place a person in a given group, by assigning a probability level to that person's belonging to each of the groups. Thus, for one person, the probabilities that he falls into each of the three groups may be 0.85, 0.09, and 0.06, respectively, and we would be fairly sure of our classifying him into the first group. But for another person, if the respective probabilities assigned are 0.24, 0.40, and 0.35, we would have to say that that person most resembles the second group, but we wouldn't be as sure because there is an almost equal probability that she could be from the last group.

C.R.A.P. DETECTORS

Example 15-1

A researcher studying a group of insomniacs and a group of normal sleepers measures the following variables on each subject: (1) sleep onset latency, (2) total sleep time, (3) total rapid eye movement (REM) time, (4) percent REM, (5) total time in stages 3 and 4, and (6) percent time in stages 3 and 4.

Question 1. How many equations will there be?

Answer. Because there are only two groups, there will be just one discriminant function, irrespective of the number of variables.

C.R.A.P. Detector XV-1

The researcher should report how "good" the discriminant function(s) is. Is it significant? How well does it classify the subjects? And so forth.

Question 2. What is the minimum number of subjects that should be in each group?

Answer. Because there are six DVs, the researcher should have at least 50 subjects in each group.

C.R.A.P. Detector XV-2

Yet again, the old 10:1 rule.

Question 3. A stepwise solution yielded four variables: latency, total sleep time, total REM, and total time in stages 3 and 4. From those data, the researcher concluded that normal sleepers and insomniacs do not differ in the *percentage* of time they spend in REM and percent deep sleep. Was this correct?

Answer. We don't know. Since percent REM and percent deep sleep are probably correlated with the other variables, it is likely that they didn't enter into the equation because they didn't add any new information. Still, the groups could have differed significantly on these variables.

C.R.A.P. Detector XV-3

Be cautious in interpreting the results of a stepwise procedure, especially in determining which variables were *not* entered. Were they really unimportant, or were they simply correlated with other variables that did enter into the equation?

Question 4. The researcher reported that 75% of the subjects were correctly classified on the basis of the equation. Can you expect results this good if you now used the equation with your patients?

Answer. No. A discriminant function always does better in "classifying" the subjects from which it was derived than in doing so with a new group. How much better is extremely difficult to determine.

C.R.A.P. Detector XV-4

The "goodness" of an equation in classifying subjects should always be tested on a "cross-validation" sample (ie, a group of new people who were not used in deriving the equation).

16

Exploratory Factor Analysis

> When many different measures have been taken on the same person, it is possible to determine if some of these scores are actually reflections of a smaller number of underlying factors. Exploratory factor analysis explores the interrelationships among the variables to discover these factors.

P*erhaps the most* widely used (and misused) multivariate statistic is factor analysis. Few statisticians are neutral about this technique. Proponents feel that factor analysis is the greatest intervention since the double bed whereas its detractors feel it is a useless procedure that can be used to support nearly any desired interpretation of the data. The truth, as is usually the case, lies somewhere in between. Used properly, factor analysis can yield much useful information; when applied blindly and without regard for its limitations, it is about as useful and informative as tarot cards. In particular, factor analysis can be used to *explore the data* for patterns, or *reduce the many variables to a more manageable number*. However, before we discuss these uses, it will be helpful to probe some of the theory of factor analysis.

CORRELATION AMONG VARIABLES

The basic assumption is that it may be possible to explain the correlation among two or more variables in terms of some underlying "factor." For example, we would see our inability to run as fast as we did last year, the aches and pains that we feel afterwards, and the nap we have to take to recuperate not as three unrelated phenomena but as all reflecting one underlying cause: we are getting older. To take another example, if we see a patient's temperature and white blood count both increasing, we say that these two

144

signs are due to one cause, namely, an infection. In the jargon of statistics, these causes are called *factors*. Factors sometimes refer to observable phenomena, but more often the factors are hypothetical constructs, such as intelligence, depression, or coping ability. We cannot measure intelligence directly; we can only infer its existence from behaviors that we hypothesize are based on it, such as school grades, the time needed to figure out a puzzle, and accuracy in defining words. Our theory states that all are influenced by this hypothetical thing we call "intelligence." If we tested a number of people and found that these three measures were correlated, we would state that they were attributable to an underlying factor of intelligence.

WHAT ARE FACTORS?

Factor analysis, then, is a technique that enables us to determine whether the variables we've measured can be explained by a smaller number of factors. (Factors, just to confuse you, are similar to what measurement people call **hypothetical constructs** and what statisticians in other contexts call **latent variables**.) The variables themselves can be individual items on a questionnaire or the scores on a number of questionnaires, depending on the study.

To see how factor analysis is done, let's assume that the Education Committee of the School of Homeopathy, Osteopathy, Veterinary Medicine, and Esthetics-Intensive Training (SHOVE-IT) has developed (yet another) form for evaluating residents. Each student is evaluated along six dimensions: Knowledge, Learning Skills, History Taking, Physical Examination, Communication Skills, and Self-Assessment. The question is, are these really six separate areas, or are they all measuring just one construct ("I like this resident"), or is the answer somewhere in between?

Just looking at the names of the six scales, we might suppose that we're tapping two sets of skills: *clinical* (History Taking, Physical Examination, and Communication Skills) and *intellectual* (Knowledge, Learning Skills, and Self-Assessment). In other words, we are postulating that students' performances in the specific skill of History Taking are determined by how much or how little they have of the underlying construct of clinical skills and that their knowledge base is dependent on the amount of the Intellectual factor. But at the same time, we're saying that each of the three scales in each skill area is also measuring something that is not captured by the other two. That is, if a person's scores on both History Taking and Physical Examination were determined solely by the underlying Clinical factor and by nothing else, then these two scores would be perfectly correlated with each other (aside from any measurement of error). To the degree that they're not perfectly correlated, there is the implication that a score on a given scale is determined partly by the factor that contributes to it (as we've said) and partly by the scale's *uniqueness* (ie, what that scale measures that other scales in that factor do not).

What we've described is depicted in Figure 16-1. We think we can explain a person's performance on the six measures by postulating a smaller number of underlying factors (in this case, two). What this figure also shows is that the Clinical factor doesn't influence the three measures that are due to the Intellectual factor, and vice versa (a highly simplified view of the world, as we'll see later). Finally, we also believe that each measure is tapping something unique (the boxes with the U's) that is not picked up by the other indices. Let's see how all this is done statistically.

DERIVING THE FACTORS

To simplify our lives a bit (and to save some paper), from now on, we'll refer to the variables by using the following notation:

X_1 = Knowledge
X_2 = Learning Skills
X_3 = Self-Assessment

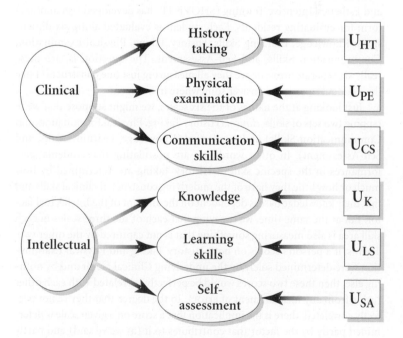

Figure 16-1 Description of factors.

X_4 = History Taking
X_5 = Physical Examination
X_6 = Communication Skills

The first step in factor analysis (as in all multivariate procedures) is to construct a **correlation matrix** showing the correlation of each variable with every other variable. Theoretically, we can stop right there and try to find groups of variables by eye. What we'd be looking for are sets of variables in which all the variables in one group correlate strongly with one another and weakly with all of the variables in the other sets. This isn't very practical, however, since the number of correlations goes up quite quickly as the number of variables increases: for n variables, there are $n(n - 1)/2$ unique correlations. Most factor analyses deal with 20 to 30 variables, meaning 190 to 435 correlations; this is far too many for any rational human being to make sense of, so we let the computer do the work for us.

What the technique does next is to construct **factors** that are similar to the linear regression equations we saw in Chapter 6. The first factor looks like the following:

$$F_1 = (Weight_1 \times X_1) + (Weight_2 \times X_2) + \ldots + (Weight_6 \times X_6)$$

Because we have six variables, we would end up with six factors, each consisting of a different set of weights for each variable. This doesn't sound like much progress; in fact, it looks like we've gone backwards, trading six scores, which we could understand, for six equations, which we can't. What is gained is the way in which the factors are constructed. The weights for the first factor are chosen so that it explains the maximum amount of the variance among the individual scores. The second factor accounts for the maximum amount of the variance that's left over, the third accounts for the maximum amount left over from the first two, and so on. If we're lucky, most of the variance will be explained (or accounted for) by only two or three factors, and we can throw away the remaining ones without losing too much information.

HOW MANY FACTORS TO KEEP

So how do we decide how many factors to keep and which ones we can toss aside? To answer this, we have to make a slight detour. In factor analysis, each variable is transformed into **standard scores**, which we saw in Chapter 2. In standard score form, each variable has a mean of zero and a standard deviation (and, therefore, a variance) of one. So the total amount of variance in the set of data is equal to the number of variables, which in this case is six. The amount of this variance that is accounted for by each factor is called its **eigenvalue**, and the sum of the eigenvalues for all of the factors equals the total variance. If we want to explain the variables in terms of a smaller number of factors, then each factor must account for the variance of at least one variable, hopefully more. So any factor with an eigenvalue of less than 1.0 is thrown out; this is called the **eigenvalue-one** or the **Kaiser-Guttman** (no relation to Kaiser Wilhelm) **criterion**. It is the most commonly used rule for deciding on the number of factors to retain and is the default option for most computer programs, but it's not the only criterion we can use.

The other widely used criterion is based on a **scree plot**, which we've shown in Figure 16-2. The factors are listed along the *x*-axis, and the eigenvalues are along the *y*-axis. This clearly shows what we discussed in the previous paragraph, namely, each succeeding factor accounts for less variance than the previous one. "Scree" is a geologic term that refers to the rubble that accumulates at the base of a cliff. Here, the "cliff" is the steep part of the graph, and the "rubble" factors are those that appear after the curve flattens out. In this example, we'd keep the first two factors and toss the remaining four.

FACTOR LOADINGS

After we've decided on how many factors to retain, using whichever criterion we (or the computer) decide to use, it's time to look at the weights that have been assigned to each variable for each factor. These are shown in Table 16-1, which is called a **factor-loading matrix** or, more commonly, a **factor**

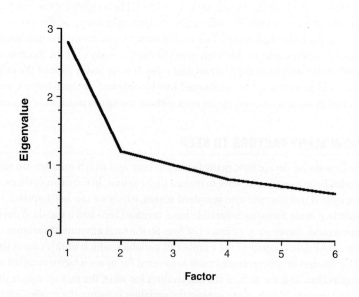

Figure 16-2 Scree plot.

Table 16-1
Factor-Loading Matrix of Six Measures

Variable	F_1	F_2
X_1	0.72	−0.10
X_2	0.78	−0.36
X_3	0.56	0.38
X_4	0.55	−0.60
X_5	0.40	0.52
X_6	0.45	0.56

matrix. It shows how much each variable correlates with, or *loads on*, each factor. In fact, each variable loads on all six factors, but we (or the computer) chose not to show the last four since they were relatively weak.

In this example, it appears as though the first factor consists of all of the variables, but most strongly, variables X_1 through X_4. The second factor consists of not only the three clinical skills measures but also two variables that also load on the first factor (X_2 and X_3). Let's digress for a moment and discuss three things: (1) when a factor loading is significant, (2) how we determine which variable goes with each factor, and (3) how we name the factor.

About the only thing statisticians agree on with regard to the significance of factor loadings is that everyone else has it wrong. For lack of any consensus, we'll adopt the criterion that to be significant, the loadings must be greater than $5.152/\sqrt{(N-2)}$.* So, if the SHOVE-IT school has assessed 150 residents, we'd be looking for loadings of 0.42 and greater (or −0.42 and less).

With regard to the second issue, a variable is assigned to the factor on which it loads most highly. Thus, because variable X_1 loads 0.72 on Factor 1 (F_1 in the table) and −0.10 on Factor 2 (F_2), we assign it to the first factor. There are times, as with variable X_4, that a variable loads on two or more factors almost equally, and it would be assigned to all. You may well ask, "How equal is 'almost equal'?" Based on all of our readings in this area and our accumulated knowledge, we can give a definitive answer: "We don't know." This is one of the many areas in statistics where experience and judgment are as important as statistical significance levels. A general rule of thumb (with the emphasis on "general") is that if one factor loading is within 0.05 of another, consider them equal.

The naming of the factors is just as arbitrary. Once you've determined which variables load on a factor, you can try to puzzle out what these variables have in common and assign a name accordingly. Some people feel that this is only an exercise in semantics and use the unimaginative (if highly

---

*If you're interested in where these strange numbers come from, see Norman GR, Streiner DL. *Biostatistics: the bare essentials.* 2nd ed. Toronto: BC Decker; 2000.

useful) names "Factor 1," "Factor 2," and so on. (Those of a classical bent use "Factor I," "Factor II," and the like, but they're just showing off.)

FACTOR ROTATION

At this point, we have completed the first two steps in factor analysis: we have extracted the factors and have kept only those that meet some criterion. We could stop at this point, but most researchers take one further step and **rotate the factors**. You may wonder why this step is necessary since the factor-loading matrix seems to tell us what we want to know. In some cases, this is true, but most of the time, and especially when we are dealing with many more variables and retained factors, there are some problems with what is called the **unrotated solution**. The first problem is that Factor 1 is usually a **general factor**, in that most of the items load significantly on it, as seems to be happening in our example. Sometimes, this is an important finding in itself, but more frequently, it is not. It simply reflects the fact that all of the measures are made on the same people, which introduces a degree of correlation among them. In most cases, we would want to focus more on the relationship among the variables after removing this "spurious" correlation within individuals. The second problem is that many of the succeeding factors are **bipolar**; that is, they have both positive and negative factor loadings. There's nothing wrong with this mathematically, but the factors are easier to interpret if all of them load in the same direction. The third difficulty is **factorial complexity**, and it reflects the fact that some variables load on two or more factors, as is the case here with variable X_4. As with bipolar factors, there is nothing wrong statistically with factorially complex variables; it is just easier to interpret the factors if they are made up of variables that load on one and only one factor. Related to this third issue, the fourth problem is that the *weights are in the middle range*, usually from 0.50 to 0.70. Again, it is harder to make sense of factors that involve a middling amount of variable A plus a so-so amount of variable B. We would much prefer the loadings to be as close to 1.0 or to 0.0 as possible; a variable either strongly loads on a factor, or it doesn't load at all.

We can illustrate these points more clearly by making a graph in which the x-axis represents Factor 1 and the y-axis represents Factor 2 and then plotting the variables. For example, variable X_1 loads 0.60 on Factor 1 and −0.25 on Factor 2, so a "1" (to indicate variable 1) is placed 0.60 units along the x-axis and 0.25 units below the origin on the y-axis. The results for all six variables are shown in Figure 16-3. This graph immediately shows the four problems. First, all the points are well to the right of the origin, indicating that they all load on Factor 1. Second, some points are above the x-axis (where the y-axis is positive), and some are below it (where the y-axis is negative), reflecting the bipolar nature of Factor 2. Third, many of the points fall toward the center of the quadrants; because they are factorially complex, they load on both factors. Fourth, few of the points are near the origin or the ends of the axes, where the loadings would be 0.0 or 1.0.

ORTHOGONAL ROTATIONAL

We can lessen the effects of these problems with a relatively simple technique called **orthogonal rotation**. Imagine that the points remain where they are, but rotate the axes clockwise about 35°, keeping them at right angles to each other. Figure 16-4 shows the new axes; the rotated Factor 1 has been relabeled F_1', and the re-drawn F_2 axis is called F_2'. Notice that this simple act of rotation has eliminated most of the problems. First, three of the variables (X_3, X_5, and X_6) lie quite close to the F_2' axis. So we've gotten around the problem of all variables loading on Factor 1. Second, most of the variables have only positive loadings. The one exception is X_4, which has a negative loading on Factor 2′; however, the magnitude of the loading is quite small. Thus, we've eliminated the problem of bipolar factors. Third, because the points lie closer to

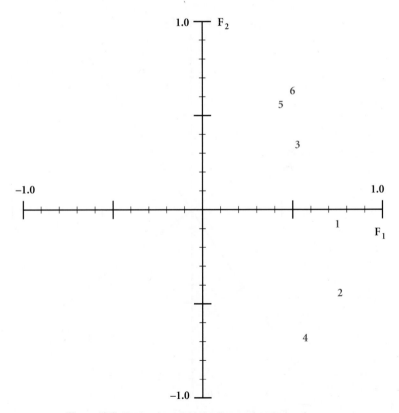

Figure 16-3 Plotting the variable loadings against the two factors.

the axes, factorial complexity is almost completely eliminated although X_1 still has a bit of it. Fourth, the points are closer to the origin of one factor and the extreme end of the other, so we've succeeded in pushing the loadings out of the middle range of values.

This rotation was relatively easy to do by eye since there were only two factors. For more complex solutions with more factors, we would be rotating axes in three-, four-, or five-dimensional space (or even higher). Fortunately, the computer can do it for us mathematically and will supply us with a **rotated factor matrix**, which is interpreted in exactly the same way as the original factor matrix.

Oblique Rotation

Before we leave this topic, it is worthwhile to mention some phrases you may encounter with respect to rotations. In introducing this topic, we said, "Rotate the axes . . . keeping them at right angles to each other," and referred

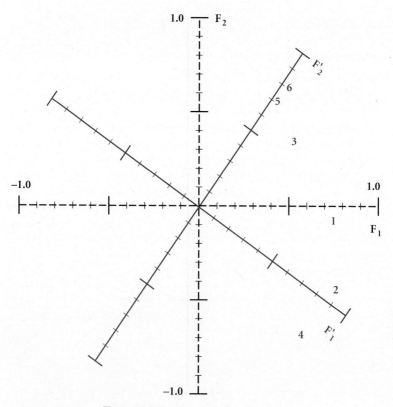

Figure 16-4 Rotation of axes from Figure 16-3.

to this type of rotation as an **orthogonal rotation**. Once in a while, a researcher may relax this condition and allow the axes to be rotated without preserving the right angles among them. This is called an **oblique rotation**. Of course, the same data could be analyzed using both methods. What is the difference between orthogonal and oblique? In the former, the factors are totally uncorrelated with one another, whereas in the latter, the angle between factors reflects their degree of correlation: the closer to 0° and the farther from 90°, the higher the correlation. An orthogonal rotation is easier to interpret, which is probably why it is preferred, but an oblique rotation often provides a more accurate reflection of reality.

Varimax Rotation

There are many ways to determine the optimal rotation, and statisticians don't agree among themselves on which is best. However, the most widely used criterion is that the rotation should maximize the variance explained by each factor. Consequently, this technique is called **varimax rotation**.

APPLICATIONS OF FACTOR ANALYSIS

Exploration of Data

Finally, let's discuss the three ways factor analysis can be used: exploration, reduction, and confirmation. In exploration (also called data dredging or a fishing expedition by those who object to this use of factor analysis), we begin with a large number of variables but no explicit hypotheses about how they hang together. In this case, we would use factor analysis to reveal patterns of interrelationships among the variables that aren't otherwise apparent. For example, we may wish to develop a battery of tests to measure cognitive recovery following a shunt operation for normotensive hydrocephaly. Not knowing beforehand which tests tap similar areas of functioning, we would begin with a large number of them and then use factor analysis to help us determine which tests cluster together; that is, we let the analysis indicate patterns within the data.

Reduction of Data

In some situations, we may want to reduce the number of variables we have on each subject for later analyses; that is, we may start off with a large number of items per subject, but for various reasons (which we'll discuss in a moment), we may want only five or six summary scores on people. Here, we could use each factor as a type of scale. If, say, 12 of the items load significantly on Factor 2, we could simply sum a person's score on those 12 variables and use this total as a new variable, effectively reducing the number of variables by 11. Often, the major reason for this use of factor analysis is to increase the subject-to-variable ratio, so that in subsequent analyses, the 10:1 rule won't be violated.

Confirmation of Hypotheses

Until about a decade or so ago, the type of factor analysis we've been describing was also used in attempts to confirm hypotheses, especially when it was used in developing scales. Since then, a more powerful variant, called **confirmatory factor analysis** (CFA), has become popular, and the more "traditional" form we discussed in this chapter is now called **exploratory factor analysis** (EFA). We'll describe CFA in Chapter 17, when we talk about path analysis and structural equation modeling. For now, suffice it to say that if you want to use EFA to confirm hypotheses, don't!

C.R.A.P. DETECTORS

Example 16-1
In order to determine which factors affect return to work following coronary bypass surgery, an investigator gives a number of cardiac, pulmonary, and psychological tests to a group of subjects, yielding a total of 35 scores.

Question 1. What is the minimum number of subjects he should have to factor-analyze the results?
Answer. If he throws all the tests into one big factor analysis, he should have at least 350 subjects.

C.R.A.P. Detector XVI-1

Factor analyses done with fewer than 100 subjects or with fewer than 10 subjects per variable (whichever is more) should be viewed with a jaundiced eye.
Question 2. Is there any way he can get around this, as there are only 50 patients a year in his town who receive the procedure?

Answer. He can factor-analyze each set of findings (cardiac, pulmonary, and psychological) independently and then later deal with the three sets of factors as if they were variables.

Question 3. Not having read this book, he throws all of the variables into the pot at the same time and reports that he ended up with six factors, with eigenvalues of 4.13, 3.87, 3.29, 2.85, 1.71, and 1.03, respectively. Would you be as ecstatic as he was about his results?

Answer. Definitely not. Because there were 35 variables, the sum of the eigenvalues for all of the factors would be 35. The six factors with eigenvalues greater than 1 account for only 48% of the variance (4.13 + . . . + 1.03 = 16.88; 16.88/35 = 0.48). That means that 52% of the variance among the 35 variables is *not* accounted for by the six factors. Ideally, the retained factors should account for at least 60%, and preferably 75%, of the variance.

C.R.A.P. Detector XVI-2

Beware of studies that don't tell you how much of the variance the factors account for; they're probably trying to hide something. If they report neither the proportion of variance nor the eigenvalues themselves (from which you can figure out the explained variance), then they are *definitely* trying to hide something.

Question 4. He reported only the eigenvalues of the retained factors and the names he assigned to them. What else is missing from the results?

Answer. Because there are so many options from which to choose when using factor analysis, he also should have reported (1) the method used to extract the principal components, (2) whether a rotation was done, (3) if so, what type of rotation, and (4) the factor-loading table itself.

Path Analysis and Structural Equation Modeling

Path analysis, an extension of multiple regression, lets us look at more than one dependent variable at a time and allows for variables to be dependent with respect to some variables and independent with respect to others. Structural equation modeling extends path analysis by looking at latent variables.

Multiple regression and factor analysis are fine as far as they go, but (as pubescent boys complain about girls) they don't go far enough. Let's first take a look at two of the shortcomings of multiple regression. First, there's only one dependent variable. There are times, though, when we'd like to see the effects of predictor variables on a number of different outcomes. For example, the three H's of Height, Hirsuteness, and Humour (ie, of the British type) may predict success in a medical faculty (a hypothesis endorsed by Norman, who is tall, bearded, and of Anglo-Saxon stock) but may also lead to an increased risk of head injuries (the belief of Streiner, who is shorter, balder, and hails from New York). Second, in multiple regression, a variable can be either a predictor (an independent variable) or an outcome (a dependent variable). A more realistic view of the world is that a given variable may be an outcome with respect to some variables but may in turn become a predictor of other variables. So, for example, head injuries may not be a direct result of bumping into low doorways (the Gerald Ford hypothesis); rather, the three H's lead to promotion to dean, which results in physical abuse by the rest of the faculty (the Streiner hypothesis). It is possible to use multiple regression to analyze these models, but it becomes quite cumbersome, with many computer runs and no easy way to synthesize the results.

PATH ANALYSIS

Types of Variables

A more direct approach to solving these problems is to use a technique called **path analysis** (PA). Over the past few years, PA has been replaced in many cases by a more sophisticated technique called **structural equation modeling** (SEM), but since PA is easier to understand and also forms the underpinnings of SEM, we'll start with PA and then graduate to the grown-up version. Although both PA and SEM are extensions of multiple regression, they rely very heavily on pictures called **path diagrams** to visualize what's going on. In fact, most of the computer programs that do PA and SEM allow you to start off with a path diagram, and they then figure out the fancy stuff. So let's begin by drawing a path diagram of a simple multiple regression, that of the three H's leading to success on the faculty, as shown in Figure 17-1.

All of the variables are represented by rectangles, and each path is represented by a straight line with an arrow head at one end. The predictor variables are joined by curved lines with arrow heads at both ends. The straight arrows (this is a geometric term, not a description of moral fiber) are the **paths**, and the curved ones represent the **correlations** among the variables. The circle with an arrow pointing to the dependent variable is the error term, called the **disturbance** term in PA and SEM and which is a part of every regression equation (and by extension, part of every PA and SEM diagram). If we want to look at another outcome variable, we simply draw another rectangle and the appropriate paths, as in Figure 17-2. In this case, we're not

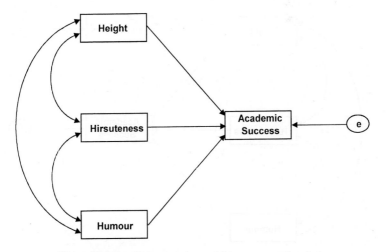

Figure 17-1 A multiple regression model drawn as a path analysis.

hypothesizing that Hirsuteness or Humour leads to head injury, so we don't draw paths connecting them.

In PA and SEM, we don't talk about "independent" and "dependent" variables. Instead, we talk about **exogenous variables** and **endogenous variables**. This shift in terminology isn't totally arbitrary. Let's take a look at the Streiner hypothesis, in which head injury is an adverse side effect of promotion and is not due directly to bumping into low objects. We can draw the model as in Figure 17-3. It's obvious that the three H's are predictor variables and that head injury is the outcome, but what do we call promotion? It's the outcome (dependent variable) with respect to the three H's, but it's the predictor (independent variable) for head injury. To avoid confusion, we say that *an exogenous variable has paths coming from it and none leading to it* (we don't count the curved arrows because they're simply describing correlations among the variables and aren't considered to be paths). Hence, the three H's are exogenous variables. Similarly, *an endogenous variable has at least one path leading to it.* So both promotion and head injury would be called endogenous variables. Note also that all endogenous variables have an error term tacked on, which corresponds to the assumption in multiple regression that the dependent variable is measured with some degree of error.

Causality and Model Building

Before we go much further, let's get a couple of myths out of the way. First, because of all those single-headed arrows, people once thought that they could use PA to prove causality; in fact, it was once referred to as "causal

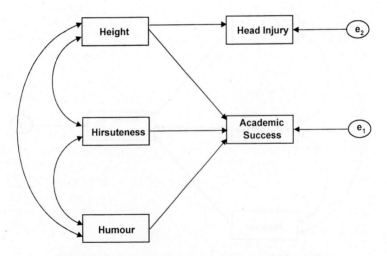

Figure 17-2 Adding a second outcome variable to the path analysis.

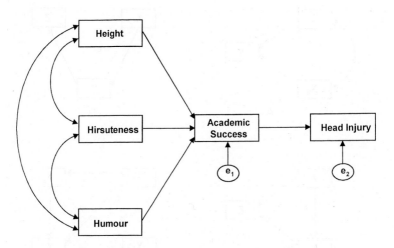

Figure 17-3 An alternative hypothesis of the relationships among the variables.

modeling". After all, if variable A has an arrow pointing toward variable B, and B points to C, then we're obviously proving that A causes B, which in turn causes C. As our kids (and those grown-ups who act like kids) would say, "Not!" The sad fact is that there are many models in which we can turn some of the arrows around to point in the opposite direction and get exactly the same results. Cause and effect can be established only through the proper research design; no amount of statistical hand waving can turn correlations into conclusions about causation.

The second myth is that we can use PA to develop theoretical models. PA and SEM are model-*testing* procedures, not model-*developing* ones. Our models should always be based on theory, knowledge, or even hunches. Modifying our model simply because it results in a more significant finding can lead us down the garden path, albeit with a very low *p* level.

Different Types of Path Models

With that out of the way, let's get back to the models themselves (all based on our extensive knowledge and solid grasp of the theories, mind you). These can be as simple or as complex as needed; in Figure 17-4, we show just a few of the many variants. Because everybody (and that includes you, now) knows that endogenous variables have error terms associated with them, we won't bother to draw them in. In Figure 17-4, A should look familiar; it shows a simple multiple regression type of model with two exogenous (X_1 and X_2) and one endogenous (Y) variable. B depicts a **mediated** model, in which Y modifies the effect of X on Z. For example, a simple version of the

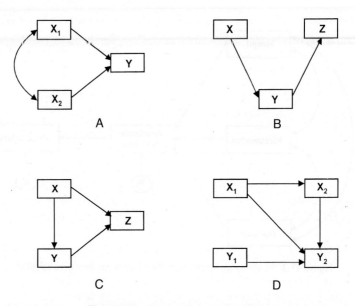

Figure 17-4 Some examples of path models.

Streiner hypothesis is that height leads to a deanship, which then leads to physical abuse from the faculty, producing head injury. In other words, there is no direct relationship between height and head injury; there is an intervening, or mediating, variable of deanship which accounts for the association. C is a bit more complex, combining elements of the two previous models. Variable X has a direct effect on variable Z but also acts on variable Y, which in turn affects Z. For example, height (variable X) may lead directly to head injury (variable Z)—the Gerald Ford hypothesis—as well as act through promotion, as in B.

Let's change the example to a real one for Figure 17-4, D. Sawyer and colleagues hypothesized that a mother's psychopathology at time 1 (X_1) would be a determinant of her pathology at time 2 (X_2) and that, similarly, the kid's pathology at time 1 (Y_1) would influence his at time 2 (Y_2). Moreover, the kid's pathology at time 2 would be also be affected by the mother's pathology at both time 1 (the path between X_1 and Y_2) and time 2 (X_2 to Y_2). Note that this model says, in essence, that his pathology at time 1 does not affect mom's either at time 1 (there's no path between Y_1 and X_1) or at time 2 (Y_1 to X_2), nor does his pathology at time 2 affect hers at time 2 (no path from Y_2 to X_2). Needless to say, if we'd had a different theoretical model of the influence of who makes who crazy, we would have drawn a different set of paths. In this example, the subscripts referred to different times. We could also use this type of model to look at different variables at the same time. For example, X_1 could be the mom's anxiety and Y_1, her depression; the variables with a subscript 2 could refer to the kid's anxiety and depression.

Recursive and Nonrecursive Models

With all of these models, the arrows go in one direction. If we start down a path, we'll never end up back where we started (we can wax philosophical at this point, commenting on how this is a model of life, but we won't). These are called **recursive models**. It may seem to make more theoretical sense, though, for the kid's anxiety to affect his depression in addition to his depression influencing his anxiety, or for the kid's mood to feed back to modify his mom's; that is, there would be an additional arrow going from Y_2 to X_2 or from Y_2 to Y_1. In this case, following a path would lead us around in circles; for some counterintuitive reason, this is called a **nonrecursive model**. The problem is that not only would we be going around in circles in the diagram, but we would also be going around in circles trying to interpret the results. The best advice we can offer about postulating a nonrecursive model is *don't try this at home*. Rather, pour yourself a stiff drink, sit back, and come up with a model that's recursive. We've known many a researcher who has tried to work with a nonrecursive model, never to be heard from again (sort of like a vice-president).

Keep It Simple, Stupid (KISS)

At first glance, it may seem as if we should have arrows from each box to every other box in Figure 17-4, D. After all, mom's depression may affect her anxiety and vice versa; we could say the same about the kid's anxiety and depression. Mom's anxiety may affect her son's anxiety and depression, and the same may be true for her depression. Finally, no parent could argue with the fact that craziness is inherited (we get it from our kids).

There are a number of reasons why having arrows from each box to every other box would be a bad idea. First of all, it would result in a nonrecursive model in spades. This would lead to the second reason, namely, that it would be next to impossible to figure out what was going on. The third reason is that there is a limit to the number of paths that can be analyzed in any one diagram; in particular, *the number of parameters is less than or equal to the number of observations*. In PA and SEM, the number of observations is not based on the sample size, but rather, on the number of variables in the model (k). The specific formula is:

$$\text{Number of observations} = [k\,(k + 1)]/2$$

Since there are four variables in Figure 17-4, D, the number of observations is $(4 \times 5) / 2 = 10$.

But how many parameters are there? That is a bit harder to figure out and requires us to expand on the purpose of running PA or SEM. The aim is to determine what affects the endogenous variables. This means that we have to determine

1. which paths are important (the straight arrows),
2. what the variances of the exogenous variables are,
3. how the exogenous variables relate to one another (the curved arrows, or covariances), and
4. what the error terms (disturbances) of the endogenous variables are.

We are *not* interested in the variances of the endogenous variables, because they are the result of the factors we just listed. So the number of parameters is *the number of paths + the number of variances of exogenous variables + the number of covariances + the number of disturbance terms.* In Figure 17-4, D, we have four paths, two variances (those for X_1 and Y_1), the covariance between these two variables, and two disturbance terms, for a total of nine parameters. Since the number of parameters is less than the number of observations, we can go ahead and analyze this model.

If we drew paths from every variable to every other variable in D, there would be twelve paths and four disturbance terms, greatly exceeding our quota and providing yet another argument against this approach. So the message is to "keep it simple, stupid"; make the model as simple as possible, but no simpler.

Was It Good for You, Too?

Now that we've postulated a model (we'll start off with the one in Figure 17-2), let's run it and see what we get. The results are shown in Figure 17-5. The numbers near the curved arrows are the correlations among the exogenous variables: Height is correlated 0.13 with Hirsuteness and −0.34 with Humour, and Hirsuteness correlates −0.31 with Humour. The numbers over the paths are the **standardized path coefficients**, which are the same as the beta weights in a multiple regression. (With most programs, we can also get the unstandardized weights, which are the *b*'s in a multiple regression.) Finally, the numbers over the endogenous variables are the squared multiple correlations, which are the R^2's in regression.

To see how well our model fits the data, we first look at the path coefficients. One question we should ask is whether the signs are correct. The signs between Height and Success, Hirsuteness and Success, and Height and Head Injury are all positive and thus in the predicted direction, so we're off to a good start. The sign between Humour and Success is also positive, which may raise some flags—who ever heard of a dean with a sense of humor? Next, the path coefficients are parameters, just as beta weights are, so that

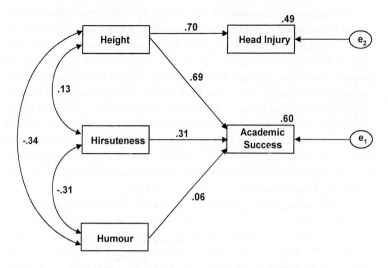

Figure 17-5 The results from running the model in Figure 17-2.

each one has its own standard error (SE). As is the case with many other tests, when we divide the parameters by their SEs, we'll get a z test. If the value of the test is greater than 1.96, then the parameter is statistically significant; otherwise, it is not. In this case, all of the path coefficients are significant with the exception of the one from Humour to Academic Success. We always had a suspicion that deans were humorless. This tells us that our hunch was wrong; there isn't any relationship between humor and being a dean, at least once height and hirsuteness are taken into account.

These tests—looking at the signs of the path coefficients and their significance levels—tell us about the individual component of the model. We can also look at the model as a whole, with a **goodness-of-fit chi-square** (χ^2_{GoF}). Everything we've learned up to now about statistical tests tells us that they're like the Hollywood concept of the bra size of the ideal female movie star: bigger is better. χ^2_{GoF} is an exception to the rule; the smaller the better. Why this sudden change of heart (or libido)? With a conventional chi-square (χ^2), we are testing the difference between our *observed* data and the *expected* findings, where the expected values are those we'd see under the null hypothesis of no association between the variables. Because we are usually aiming to demonstrate that there is an association, we want the observed values to differ from the expected one, and the more they differ, the stronger the association and the larger the value of χ^2. However, with a χ^2_{GoF}, we are testing the difference between the *observed data* and our *hypothesized model*. Because we hope that our proposed model does fit the data, we don't want to see too much difference; in fact, the ideal would be to have no difference between the two.

The degrees of freedom for χ^2_{GoF} equal the number of observations minus the number of parameters. This further reinforces the principle of KISS; the simpler the model, the more degrees of freedom there are to play with and the larger the value of χ^2 we can tolerate. There are a couple of problems with χ^2_{GoF}, though. First, it's greatly affected by the sample size of the study. If the sample size is low, then the SEs are large and it will be hard to detect a difference between the model and the data, even if the model is a poor description of the relationships among the variables. Conversely, if the sample size is too large, then even small differences between the model and the data will result in statistical significance. Second, a nonsignificant χ^2_{GoF} doesn't mean that there may not be a better model, one that fits the data even more closely; it simply means "close enough."

Finally, as we said before, we cannot draw conclusions about causality from the model, even if χ^2_{GoF} is not significant. For example, we can postulate a model in which Hirsuteness leads to Humour (Figure 17-6, a), based on the supposition that men with hair are laughing at those who are more follically challenged (women aren't so crass). If we reverse the direction of the path between Hirsuteness and Humour (see Figure 17-6, b), we end up with a bizarre model in which laughing causes hair to grow *and with exactly the same value of* χ^2_{GoF}. So, simply because the model fits doesn't mean it's right.

STRUCTURAL EQUATION MODELING

Measured and Latent Variables

Let's go back and look at the variables we examined with PA and how they were measured. Height is easy; we just put a long ruler next to the person and read off the number. Academic success is also easy; it's an ordinal scale

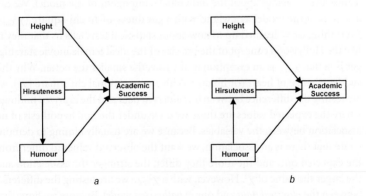

Figure 17-6 Both models have the same Goodness-of-Fit Index.

of lecturer, assistant professor, and so on, up to university president (which, unfortunately, ignores who really runs the university, namely, all of those secretaries who control who gets to meet with whom, what meetings get called or cancelled, and which promotion dossiers get misplaced at inconvenient times). We can measure hirsuteness by actually counting hairs or by using some global assessment, and humor can be assessed by using a laugh meter (so beloved by old television shows) or colleagues' ratings. No matter how they're scored, these are all **measured** variables; that is, variables that are observed directly by physical measurement (eg, height, blood pressure, serum rhubarb) or on a scale such as a written test of one sort or another. For a number of reasons that we'll get into, it is often preferable to use **latent** variables in our models in addition to or instead of measured ones. We've encountered latent variables before, but they went by another name. When we discussed factor analysis, we said that a number of variables or items may be observed manifestations of an underlying factor. A **factor** in factor analysis is called a **latent variable** in SEM and other statistical procedures—same idea, just a different name. To repeat, a factor or latent trait is an unseen construct, such as intelligence or anxiety or depression, that is responsible for the correlations among the measured variables that we do see. For example, if we note that a medical student interacts warmly with patients, treats the nurses with respect, and acknowledges the superior wisdom and knowledge of her supervisors, we say that she has good "interpersonal skills," but (1) we don't see interpersonal skills directly, only its manifestations, and (2) we assume that warmth, respect, and deference are all correlated with one another. We can show that, as in Figure 17-7.

There are a couple of things to note about this diagram. First, the SEM convention is to use an oval to indicate a latent variable. Second, note the direction of the arrows: they come *from* the latent variable *to* the measured ones. This is important; it reflects the fact that the measured variables are due to or are the result of the latent factor. Finally, each of the measured variables has a circle with a *D* inside. Because the measured variables in this case are endogenous (they have arrows pointing to them from Interpersonal Skills), they need an error term. In multiple regression, we denote this with an *e*; in factor analysis, we refer to it as the variable's *uniqueness*; and in SEM, we use a *D* to stand for **disturbance**. Yet again, it's exactly the same idea in each case, but with a different term in order to confuse and mystify.

Factor Analysis and SEM

Let's continue to explore the similarity of SEM to factor analysis because this will help us later in discussing the power of this technique. If we used SEM on the (fictitious) data for Figure 17-7, what we would get is shown in Figure 17-8. The numbers over the paths from Interpersonal Skills to the three

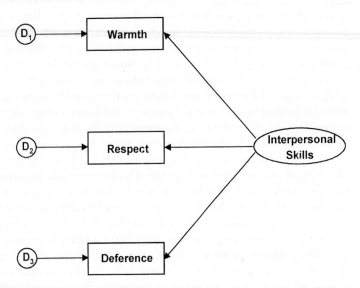

Figure 17-7 An example of a factor (or latent variable) with three measured variables.

measured variables are the path coefficients. These are identical in both meaning and value to the **factor loadings** we'd get if we ran a factor analysis on these data, and the numbers from the disturbance terms to the variables are identical to the **uniqueness** terms. In factor analysis:

$$(\text{Factor loading})^2 + (\text{uniqueness})^2 = 1$$

which translates into SEM terms as:

$$(\text{Path coefficient})^2 + (\text{disturbance})^2 = 1$$

So, for Warmth, for example, $(0.543)^2 + (0.840)^2 = 1.00$. To find the correlation between any two variables, we multiply their path coefficients (or factor loadings). The correlation between Warmth and Respect is therefore $0.840 \times 0.797 = 0.67$.

The Advantages of Latent Variables

Why make such a big deal over our ability to use latent variables in SEM? There are a couple of reasons, both of which are very powerful. First, we are often in a situation where we have a number of different measures of the same construct, none of which are ideal. For instance, if we are doing a study of rheumatoid arthritis, there are a number of lousy outcomes: joint count,

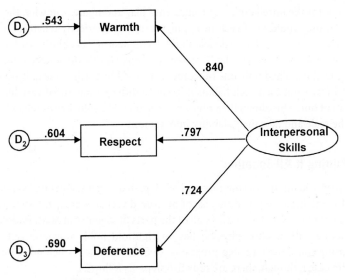

Figure 17-8 The results of analyzing Figure 17-7.

duration of morning stiffness, sedimentation rate, and so on. Using them all presents many problems, such as what to conclude if some improve and some get worse, inflation of the alpha level because of the numerous tests that must be run, different measurement scales for each, and so forth. (Note that this is a different situation from looking at academic success and head injury as outcomes in Figure 17-2; they are in separate realms, and there is no theoretical reason to combine them.) SEM allows us to consider them simultaneously, as various measured variables reflecting the latent variable of Outcome.

The second reason has to do with measurement theory. Each of the measured variables is unreliable to varying degrees; that is, two independent raters will disagree with one another in assessing how many joints are inflamed, and two successive laboratory tests will give different values for the sedimentation rate. This puts an upper limit to how highly any other variable can correlate with them. So even if we make the outrageous assumption that nonsteroidal anti-inflammatory drug dose correlates −1.0 with joint count, the correlation we'd find in a study will not approach this because counting inflamed joints is such an unreliable measure. The result of unreliability is that we underestimate the relationships among variables or the effects of an intervention.

By considering them as simply different measures of the same construct, SEM can determine the reliability of each variable and then "disattenuate" the reliabilities. In plain English, this means that an equation that compensates for the unreliability is brought into play and figures out what the correlations would be if each of the measures were perfectly reliable. (If you want more of the dreary details about disattenuating reliabilities with nothing more than a hand calculator, see our book *Health Measurement Scales*.) In fact, if we had only one outcome scale, we'd be further ahead if we split it in two and used each half as if it were a different measured variable of a latent one. This allows the program to calculate the split-halves reliability of the scale and take the reliability into account.

Putting It All Together

We've laid out the various pieces of SEM: path diagrams, measured variables, disturbance terms, and the use of measured variables as manifestations of latent ones. Now let's see how all of the parts fit together in SEM. Buddhism (along with nuclear physics) has an eightfold noble way, and self-help groups have their 12-step programs; so SEM can't be far behind. To make life easier, though, there are only five steps, as follows:
1. Model specification
2. Model identification
3. Estimation
4. Test of fit
5. Respecification

Model Specification

Model specification, which is also called the **measurement model**, consists of specifying the relationships among the latent variables and determining how the latent variables will be measured. It is probably the most important step, as well as the most difficult one. It's the most crucial step because everything else follows from it; specify the model incorrectly or choose the wrong measured variables to reflect the latent ones, and there's little that can save you down the road. It's the most difficult step because the computer can't help at this stage; you actually have to think on your own. You specify the model, based on your knowledge of the field, on your reading of the literature, or on theory. So let's go ahead and expand our model to reflect a more sophisticated understanding of the academic world.

First, we recognize that height alone doesn't capture the whole picture. Who cares if you're as tall as Wilt Chamberlain, if you look like a wimp, or tip the scales at 150 kilos (that's 331 pounds for those of you in the United States, Liberia, and Myanmar). So we'll use Height as one measured variable, along with body build index (BBI), to reflect the latent variable of Stature. Second, Hairiness, at least for men, can consist of head hair (measured on a five-point ordinal scale of full / thinning / fringe / absent / replaced) and facial hair (rabbinical / Vandyke / mustache / none). Third, Humour also has two parts, both measured on seven-point Likert scales: (1) Tells Good Jokes and (2) Laughs at My Jokes.

Turning to the consequences of these attributes, we recognize that academic rank only partly captures our true worth. Our colleagues envy us not for our titles but for the number of talks we give in foreign countries, best measured by Air Miles. And finally, we can capture Head Injury by scores on a memory test and the number of circular indentations. Putting this all together, we get the model shown in Figure 17-9.

Model Identification

The rule that we stated for PA—that the number of parameters cannot exceed, and ideally should be much less than, the number of observations—also holds for SEM. As before, the best way to limit the number of parameters is to leave out paths that aren't postulated by our theory, knowledge, or hunches. In SEM, though, we have to go a bit further and place limits on some of the paths and variables. For example, there are two paths leading from Stature to its measured variables, Height and BBI. One of those paths must be set equal to 1. To understand why, we'll use an analogy. Let's say we want to solve the equation:

$$a = b + c$$

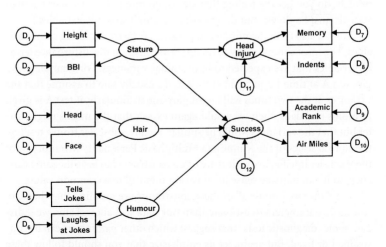

Figure 17-9 An expanded structural equation model of Figure 17-2.

If we know that $a = 10$, then what are the values of b and c? The answer is that there are literally an infinite number of possibilities: $b = 1$ and $c = 9$, $b = 2$ and $c = 8$, $b = -832.8$ and $c = 842.8$, and so on. The equation is solvable only if we limit the values that b and c can assume, and we can do this in one of two ways. The first way is to **fix** either b or c to some specific value. For example, if we say that b is equal to 7.3, then we can solve for c. The second way is to **constrain** b and c by saying, for instance, that they're equal to one another, in which case both have the value of 5.

This gives us three types of variables:

1. **Free** variables, which can assume any value and whose values are determined by the equations of SEM
2. **Fixed** variables, which are assigned a specific value by the user
3. **Constrained** variables, which are unknown (like free variables) but are set equal to some other parameter

To solve the equations, *one path from a latent variable to its measured variables must be fixed.* It doesn't matter which one is fixed or what the fixed value is. If the reliabilities of the measured variables are known beforehand, it's best to fix the one with the highest reliability. By convention and for the sake of simplicity, the fixed path is given a value of 1. We can use any other value, and although doing so won't change the values of the standardized path coefficients, it will alter the values of the unstandardized coefficients.

For the same reason, we fix the paths leading from the disturbance terms to the exogenous variables to be 1. Actually, we can fix either the path or the variance of the error term itself (in the same way that we can fix either b or c in the equation). In reality, though, we rarely know the error variance ahead of time, so the path is the term we fix. (Between "fixing" paths and altering models, do you get the feeling that we sound more like veterinarians than statisticians? So do we. But don't worry; we don't spay any variables.)

We can also limit the number of parameters by constraining some variables. The most common way to do this is to constrain the disturbance terms of variables that are expected to have similar variances. For example, if we give test A at time 1 and again at time 2, it's usually safe to assume that the variances at the two times will be roughly equal. Similarly, if test A is given to moms and dads, then we would again expect that the means might differ but that the variances would be similar. Finally, subscales from a test (eg, the clinical scales of the Minnesota Multiphasic Personality Inventory or of the Wechsler intelligence scales) are often constructed to have the same variance, so it would make sense to constrain them all to a common value.

Even after we impose all of these constraints, we may find that there are still more parameters to estimate than our data will allow. Later, we'll discuss some "diagnostic tests" that suggest which other parameters can be constrained or fixed. But again, let us emphasize that you should follow these suggestions *only if they make sense* on the basis of theory, knowledge, or previous research and not simply because they improve the statistics. (However, just to be sure, we'll repeat the message later on.) At this point, our model looks like Figure 17-10.

Estimation

Now that we've specified the model and fixed or constrained some of the paths or variances, the fun begins; we're ready to get down to business and estimate the parameters. But as we've seen so often with sophisticated techniques, we're again faced with the issue of many different approaches. And as before, if one method was clearly superior to the others, it would have won the Darwinian battle and survived while the others became footnotes. This book has no footnotes, indicating that all are still alive and kicking.

The major advantage to the **unweighted least squares** approach is that it doesn't make any assumptions about the underlying distributions of the variables. This means that we don't have to worry about normality, skewness, or any other nasty facts of life. So why isn't this approach king of the mountain? Its limitation—and it's a big one—is that the results are dependent on the scale of measurement. So if we measured height in centimeters instead of inches, or if Air Miles were awarded on the basis of kilometers rather than miles flown, we'd get very different results. Needless to say, this is a most undesirable property except in a few areas in which there is universal agreement about the variables (eg, lab medicine, if the Americans ever get around to adopting SI units), so this method is only rarely used.

The **weighted least squares** approach gets around this limitation and retains the desirable property of being distribution free. But even by the

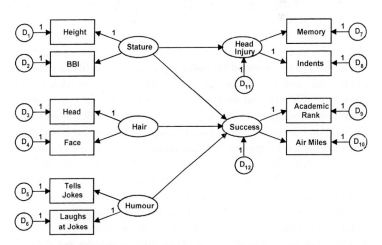

Figure 17-10 The model in Figure 17-9 after imposing constraints.

standards of SEM, in which large sample sizes are the norm (as we'll discuss later on), this one is a pig (oops— slipping back into veterinarian language), limiting its use in most situations.

So by default, most people use the **maximum likelihood** method. It is not dependent on the scale of measurement and doesn't make outrageous demands for subjects. The problem is that it requires multivariate normality (ie, all the variables are normal when looked at together), so it shouldn't be used with ordinal scales or with measures that are highly skewed. Some advanced programs, such as LISREL, have "front end" programs that can take ordinal or skewed data and transform them into forms that can be used, and similar fixes will likely become more common with other programs in the future.

Test of Fit

Now that we've run the model, it's time to ask the question, "How good was it for you?" With PA, we did three things: we looked at the signs of the coefficients; determined if they were statistically significant; and used the χ^2_{GoF} test to look at the model as a whole. We do the same things with SEM, but (as befits a more advanced technique) we have a plethora of other indices. And you guessed it—there are so many because none is ideal.

As we said in the context of PA, the major problem with the χ^2_{GoF} test is its sensitivity to the normality of the data and to the sample size: too many subjects, and it's always significant; too few subjects, and it never is. Its major attraction is that, of all of the fit indices used in SEM, it's the only one that has a test of significance associated with it. As a *rough* rule of thumb, you want χ^2_{GoF} to be nonsignificant and χ^2_{GoF} / *df* to be less than 2.

The other indices can be grouped into two main categories: **comparative fit** and **variance explained**. With one exception (which we'll mention), all are scaled to be between 0 and 1, with larger numbers indicating a better fit and with a minimum criterion of 0.90. The most common comparative fit index is the **Normed Fit Index** (NFI), which tests if the model differs from the null hypothesis that none of the variables are related to each other. The problem is that the more parameters you toss into the model, the better it becomes, just as with multiple regression, in which every variable entered into the equation increases R^2. The drawback is that if you put the scores from a new sample into the same equation, you'd be less and less likely to get as high a value of R^2 as the number of variables increases. So, a variant of the NFI, called (with an amazing lack of imagination) the **Normed Fit Index 2** (NFI 2), penalizes you for your lack of parsimony.

There are literally dozens of other comparative fit indices, but they're all based on the same ideas: (1) how much the model deviates from the null hypothesis of no relationships, and (2) shrinking the index as the number of variables increases.

The most common measure based on the amount of variance accounted for in the model is the **Goodness-of-Fit Index** (GFI). Fortunately, its formula is too complicated to burden you with (or for our understanding). As would be expected, there's a variant of it, called the **Adjusted Goodness-of-Fit Index** (AGFI), which adjusts for the number of parameters (the fewer the better) and the sample size (the more the better) with an even more complicated formula.

Somewhat different from these is **Akaike's Information Criterion** (AIC). It's different in three ways. First, it's not scaled between 0 and 1 but between a small value (which is often over 100) and a much bigger value. Second, it's the only measure in which smaller is better. Finally, it's not any good for looking at a single model since nobody (including Akaike) knows what a decent value is. It finds its place in comparing models; the one with the lower value has a better fit with the data.

How do we interpret the results, especially when a typical output may include 20, 30, or more fit indices? First, stick with the NFI 2 and AGFI. If they are both over 0.90, and the χ^2_{GoF} is not significant, you're golden; go ahead and publish. If the indices are above 0.90 but the χ^2_{GoF} is significant, look to see if your sample size may be "too large" (about which more later). If only some of the indices are over 0.90 and the χ^2_{GoF} is significant, you've got problems. The model is of borderline significance and could probably stand some tuning up, which we'll now discuss.

Respecification

"Respecification" is a fancy term for trying to improve your model to get a better fit. Bear in mind that there are a couple of tests that tell you whether some variables or paths are unnecessary or if paths or covariances should be added. *There are no tests to tell you if you forgot to include some key variables.* Misspecification due to omitted variables is probably the major cause of a bad fit in PA, SEM, multiple regression, and all other multivariable techniques. Most often, by the time you've reached this stage of the analysis, it's too late because the variables weren't collected in the first place. The only way to avoid this is to have a firm grounding in the theory and the literature so that the study captures the important information. However, don't go overboard and measure everything that moves; as we've discussed, there's a limit to how many variables you can cram into one model.

The **Lagrange multiplier tests** tell you how much the model could be improved if fixed or constrained variables were allowed to be free (in other words, if parameters were added to the model). Conversely, the **Wald test** shows the effects of deleting parameters from the model, such as by removing paths or constraining variables. We'll state again (we promise, for the last time) that you should not blindly follow the recommendations of these tests simply to improve the model. Whether or not to free a parameter or to add or drop a covariance term *must be based on your theory and knowledge*; SEM is a model-testing procedure, not a model-building one.

Sample Size

Path analysis and SEM are *very* hungry when it comes to sample size. Sample size is extremely difficult to figure out ahead of time by using exact equations since we often don't have the necessary information about the strength of the relationships among the variables. If we go by our old standby of 10 subjects, bear in mind that in this case, it's 10 subjects *per parameter*, not per variable. In SEM, each measured variable usually has three parameters: its path coefficient, its variance, and the disturbance term. Even if you have only a few parameters, though, there should be a minimum of 100 subjects. On the other hand, if you have far more than 10 subjects per parameter, be forewarned that the χ^2_{GoF} may be statistically significant, even if the model fits relatively well.

What It All Means

We can interpret the results of an SEM from two perspectives: the *measurement model* and the *model as a whole*. The measurement model part pertains to each latent variable and its associated measured variables, and there are three questions that can be asked: (1) How well do the measured variables reflect the latent one? (2) Are some observed variables better than others? and (3) How reliable is each measured variable? Each latent variable is a minifactor analysis, so we can go back and remove variables that don't seem to be doing much except adding error variance. Once we've derived a set of measured variables that work well, we can turn our attention to the model as a whole to see how well it fits the data. Are there some latent variables that don't have significant paths to others or (even worse) have significant paths but with the wrong sign?

Factor Analysis Redux

In the previous chapter, we said that hypothesis *testing* is better done with SEM and that the traditional form of factor analysis is more *exploratory* (hence its back-formed "new" name, **exploratory factor analysis**). Let's expand on that a bit. In exploratory factor analysis (EFA), we throw all of the variables into the pot, close our eyes, press the right button (which may be difficult with our eyes closed, but that's a different issue), and see what comes out. We can look at the factor structure and ask whether it matches some preconceived idea or what we expected. The problems with this way of going about things are that (1) the answer is most often, "well, sort of," and (2) the analysis doesn't take our preconceptions into account.

What we've been doing in the measurement model phase of SEM is a bit different. We are stating explicitly that a given latent variable is best reflected by these three or four measured ones and then seeing if our supposition is confirmed. You shouldn't be surprised to learn that this is called **confirmatory factor analysis**. In fact, we can have increasingly more stringent criteria for confirmation. At the lowest level, we can simply posit that certain measured variables are associated with a latent one; next, we can specify what we think the values of the path coefficients should be; and finally, we can even indicate the hypothesized variances of the variables. This gives us a powerful set of tools for comparing groups. For example, we can run an EFA on an English version of a scale and then see how well a translated version compares. First, by "confirming" the model derived from the English version with the translated one, we would determine whether the same items load on the same factors. If they do, we can then see if the items load to the same degree by testing the model using the loadings from the English version as the path coefficients and, finally, by inserting the variances from the original. If the translated model still fits after all these restrictions, then we can be fairly confident that the two versions are comparable. Similarly, we can derive a model of the relationships among variables on women and see if the same model applies to men or to any other groups.

SUMMARY: SOME CAUTIONS

PA and SEM are very powerful techniques. This means that they are ideally suited for leading you down the garden path if you're not careful. First, despite their earlier name of *causal modeling*, they cannot prove causation; they can refute it if the model doesn't fit, but all they can do is offer support if the model does fit. Second, the most common approach, maximum likelihood, is sensitive to deviations from normality. You'll get results, but they probably won't be an accurate reflection of what's going on. Finally, PA and SEM are model-testing procedures, not model-building ones. (Okay, so we lied, but the message is worth repeating.)

C.R.A.P. DETECTORS

Example 17-1

To test if people get mental disorders from their children, some researchers measure the following in 50 kids: (1) the cleanliness of the bedroom, (2) the number of times "Aw, must I?" is said in a 1-hour block, and (3) the interval between when the kid should be home and when the kid actually arrives. In the mothers, the researchers measure (1) the amount of Prozac taken each day, (2) the number of times "You're driving me crazy" is said in a 1-hour block, and (3) the amount of time spent watching game shows (as a surrogate for catatonia).

Question 1. What's the maximum number of parameters there can be in the model?

Answer. Since there are six variables, there can be a maximum of $(6 \times 7) / 2 = 21$ parameters.

Question 2. What should the sample size be?

Answer. This is hard to know without seeing the model itself, but if the number of parameters is anywhere near the limit, a sample size of 200 would be necessary to get reproducible results.

Question 3. The authors said that there was a significant improvement in the model when they added a covariance term between cleanliness and lateness arriving home. Should they have?

Answer. If there's no theoretical justification for adding that term, it shouldn't be there.

Question 4. How else can they improve their model?

Answer. Because all of the kid variables and all of the parent variables are likely tapping the same thing (teenage behavior and maternal reaction), it may be better to create two latent variables and use the measured variables to define them.

Question 5. The authors conclude that since the model fits well, it proves that the direction of causality is from the child to the parent.

Answer. Absolutely not. You cannot use PA or SEM to prove causality. The model may work just as well (or even better) with some of the arrows turned around. Are they right?

Question 6. Because it fits so well and because there are no genetic variables in it, the model demonstrates that psychiatric disorders are due solely to environmental factors. Is this a valid conclusion?

Answer. You can't test what ain't there. There's no way of knowing how much the model may be improved even further by adding genetic factors or other variables.

Cluster Analysis

> In factor analysis, we determined whether different variables can be grouped together in some specific way. With cluster analysis, we examine whether people (or animals, diagnoses, or any other entities) can be grouped on the basis of the similarities.

In Chapter 16, we discussed how factor analysis can be used to *find interrelationships among variables.* In this chapter, we examine a class of techniques, collectively termed cluster analysis, that attempts to *find interrelationships among objects.* (Despite objections from humanists and others, people are referred to as "objects," as are animals, psychiatric diagnoses, or geographic areas. This is just jargon, not a philosophical statement.) There are two major (and many minor) classes of cluster analytic techniques, with about a dozen different methods in each class, and the number is still growing. Complicating the issue even further, various authors use completely different names to refer to the same method. We can't begin to mention, much less discuss, all of these different techniques, so refer to some of the books and articles referenced in the Bibliography if you want to plow your way through this field.

METHODS OF CLASSIFYING DATA

Cluster analysis began with biologists' attempts to classify similar animals and plants into groups and to distinguish them from other groups of animals and plants. For a long time, this was done by the individual taxonomist (that is, someone who classifies, not an agent for the Revenuers) on the basis of his perception of anatomic and morphologic similarities and differences. Needless to say, this led to many disputes among taxonomists because what

177

was an obvious similarity to one person was just as obviously a difference to another. In 1963, Sokal and Sneath wrote *Principles of Numerical Taxonomy*, which attempted to introduce some mathematical rigor to the field. However, instead of bringing people together (which, after all, is one of the aims of classification), it served to broaden the points of argument and to introduce yet another area of disagreement. Now, people were fighting over the best numerical technique and battling those who maintained that the intuitive process of classification could not be reduced to "mindless" computer algorithms.

So, what is all this debate about? As you may have already deduced, "clustering" and "classifying" are synonymous terms that refer to (1) the grouping of objects into sets on the basis of their similarities and (2) the differentiating between sets on the basis of their differences. For example, all clinicians "know" that they can classify their patients on bases other than diagnostic: patients who come in only when they're on death's doorstep; those who make appointments every time a new pimple appears, convinced that it is the first sign of melanoma; those who blindly follow any advice given; those who won't take their medications, no matter how often they're told to do so; and so on. How would a clinician go about classifying these patients on a more objective basis?

Before beginning, the investigator must decide what he or she thinks the world is actually like because this will dictate which of the two major classes of cluster analysis to use: hierarchical methods or partitioning methods. This choice is a very important one because analyzing data with the wrong method will most likely yield some results, but they may be quite discrepant from "reality." As the name implies, "hierarchical clustering methods" end up looking like trees, such as those drawn by zoologists to classify animals. The kingdom of animals is subdivided into various phyla, which in turn branch into different classes, and so on down the line until each animal can be uniquely placed within its particular species or subspecies. The underlying assumption is that each subspecies is unique but that all of the subspecies within a given species have something in common. Similarly, the species are different from each other, but we can move up to a higher level of organization, the genus, in which all of the member species are somehow related. So if our investigator chose this method, it would reflect an implicit or explicit belief that there is a *hierarchy of patient types*. Patients can, for example, be subdivided into two groups, namely, the abusers and the good guys. Each of these groups can be further divided in two, as in dividing abusers into overusers and underusers. At the end, there will be as many little groups as patient types, all arranged in a hierarchical manner.

Partitioning methods, on the other hand, assume that each cluster is different from every other cluster, and there is no higher level of organization that can group the cluster together. Among major diagnostic groupings, the carcinomas form one cluster, quite distinct from the arteriosclerotic diseases, and both of these differ from the hemopoietic disorders. The choice of this method would reflect a "model" of the world in which the chronic complaining patient would have nothing in common with the noncompliant ones, who in turn are different from the hypochondriacs.

Hierarchical Methods

Because it is the easier method to understand, let's begin by discussing the hierarchical method. As a first step, the investigator would record various measures from or about each patient. These may include age, sex, marital status, number of visits in the past 12 months, proportion of visits in which nothing was found, index of the severity of illness at each presentation, and anything else deemed relevant. We begin by constructing a matrix, where each entry is an **index of similarity** between patients. The problem at this point is to decide what we mean by similar or dissimilar.

The earliest similarity index was the correlation coefficient in which, instead of correlating two variables across all subjects, two subjects were correlated across all variables. You may still run across the terms "Q-type correlation," "Q-type factor analysis," and "inverse factor analysis," which refer to this way of correlating people and then factor-analyzing the matrix. This was the original "cluster analysis." Articles that use this term should be at least 20 years old, or the author hasn't kept up with the times. There are many theoretical problems associated with correlating two subjects across variables as an index of similarity. For example, we normally interpret a correlation as meaning, "On the basis of subject 1's score on text X, I would predict that his score on test Y would be …" This makes sense because X and Y are related and because the same person is taking both tests. If we turn this around and correlate across tests, we would have to say that, "On the basis of subject 1's responses, I would predict that subject 2 will do …" However, unlike two tests done by the same person, subject 1 is independent of subject 2, so that the logic breaks down completely.

Moreover, the correlation coefficient cannot even tell us if the *pattern of* scores on the various tests is similar from one person to another. Let's take a look at Figure 18-1. In A, the two people have parallel profiles, differing only in level. As we would expect, the correlation is +1.0. But the correlations for B and C are also +1.0 because the scores for one person are related linearly to the other person's scores in each case. For these and many other reasons, the correlation coefficient isn't (or, at least, shouldn't be) used as an index of similarity.

In its place, similarity is now measured by some index of the *distance* between the sets of points. The difficulty here, as with many multivariate procedures, is an embarrassment of riches. There are probably three dozen

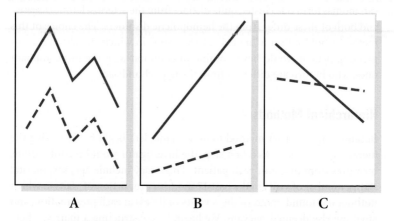

Figure 18-1 Various ways two curves could yield a correlation of +1.0.

different indices, ranging from the simple measurement of the distances between the raw scores called the "unstandardized Euclidian distance" to highly sophisticated techniques with such forbidding names as the "Minkowski metric," "Mahalanobis' D^2," or the "city block metric." All of the measures try to do the same thing, namely, to come up with one number that expresses how far apart or how dissimilar two sets of scores are from one another. If one method were clearly superior to all of the others, there would be only one measure around. The plethora of indices indicates that each method has its limitations and that each index makes realistic or tenable assumptions. More unfortunately, the various indices can give rise to quite different solutions.

For the sake of simplicity, assume the investigator collected data from only six patients, whom we'll call A through F. (Naturally, by this point, you know enough that *you* would never settle for such a small sample size, especially with so many variables.) We start by calculating our 6 × 6 similarity matrix. If we find that B and E have the highest similarity index, we would draw a line connecting them (Figure 18-2). We consider B and E together to be one group and go back to our similarity matrix, which now is of size 5 × 5, to find the next highest index.

We may find that C and F are most similar, and we would draw this as shown in Figure 18-3. The lines connecting C and F are longer than those connecting B and E because C and F are more dissimilar to each other than B is dissimilar to E.

In essence, the shorter the horizontal lines, the more similar the objects. We now have four "objects" to group: two objects of one member each (A and D) and two objects that have two members each (BE and CF). If our next highest similarity index reveals that BE is most similar to A, our tree graph, or *dendogram,* is as shown in Figure 18-4.

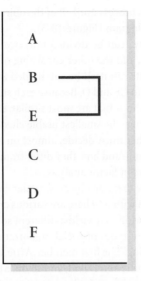

Figure 18-2 Step 1 of the dendogram.

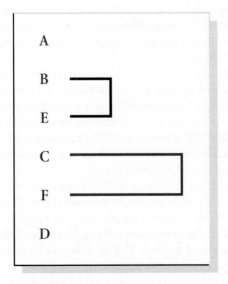

Figure 18-3 Step 2 of the dendogram.

We continue this process until all of the objects are joined, as, for example, in the final dendogram (Figure 18–5).

Thus, the "family" can be divided into two groups: one consisting of patients A, B, and E, and the other consisting of patients C, F, and D. The first group of patients can itself be subdivided into two groups, A and BE, as can the second, into CF and D. Because each step of the process combines the two objects or groups that are most similar, each branch always has two twigs. In real situations, the smallest usable cluster will contain at least five objects. The researcher must decide, almost on a clinical basis, what these objects have in common and how they differ from the other sets. This is similar to naming factors in factor analysis.

How do we know that one object is similar enough to another object or group to be included with it? There are various criteria with which to work, and again, each criterion may yield a different solution. These methods are analogous to different types of social organizations. One method is like a club that's just forming. The first member, Artie, asks his friend Bob to join. Bob then invites Charlie and David, and so on. Meanwhile, a second, parallel club is being formed in a similar manner, with Stuart asking Tom, who then asks Urquhart (*you* try to think of a name beginning with "U") and Victor. This method requires simply that the newcomer be similar to at least one member of the already existing group. The advantage of this relatively lax criterion is that every person usually ends up in a group. However, we often find that there is a lot of diversity among objects within a group. Object C may join group AB because it is similar to B, and then D may be added because it resembled C; but A and D may be quite dissimilar to one another. This criterion is called **single linkage** because the object has to link up with only a single member. It is also referred to as the nearest-neighbor or space-contracting method.

We can avoid this problem by being more exclusive and stipulating that the proposed new member can be blackballed if it differs from *any* of the previous members. This results in a country club atmosphere in which there are nice tight groupings of almost identical members but also a lot of outsiders that have little in common with the members or with each other. The term for this criterion is **complete linkage** (a.k.a. furthest-neighbor, space-distorting, and four or five other aliases).

Given these two extremes, it is almost superfluous to say that someone has staked out a middle ground. In this case, it consists of comparing the newcomer with the average of the groups and joining it to the group whose mean is most similar to its scores, yielding the **average linkage**, or **UPGMC**, or **nearest centroid method**. This is analogous to joining one political group as opposed to another. You join the one whose beliefs are most similar to your own, knowing that there will be some degree of heterogeneity of people, who will differ from you to some degree along some dimensions.

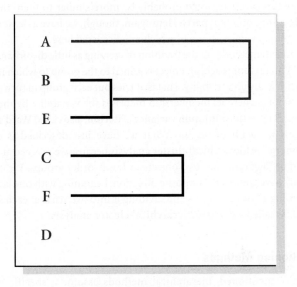

Figure 18-4 Step 3 of the dendogram.

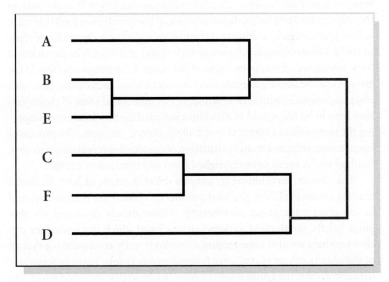

Figure 18-5 Final step of the dendogram.

Despite this diversity, you'd probably be more similar to them than to the people from a different party. Here again, though, we have at least four ways of defining "average," none of which are discussed here.

A fourth method is in the tradition of creating as little disturbance as possible. With this approach, an object is joined to the group to which it adds the least within-group variability. That is, it tries out each group in turn and sticks with the one where its membership increases the variability by the smallest amount. This is the **minimum variance criterion**, also called Ward's method.

Now for a bit of jargon. What we have just described is called an **agglomerative hierarchical cluster analysis** because we proceed at each step to join or "agglomerate" two objects or lower-order groups. We could just as easily have gone in the opposite direction, beginning with one large group containing all of the objects and dividing it into two parts at each step. This would be called a **divisive hierarchical cluster analysis**.

Partitioning Methods

As we've mentioned, hierarchical methods assume a specific model of patient taxonomy, namely, that there is a hierarchical arrangement of patient types. If the researcher assumed a different model, one that assumed that each type is unique, he would then choose a different brand of cluster analysis, the **partitioning method**.

Unlike hierarchical methods, the partitioning models do not start off with a similarity matrix. Instead, the investigator makes a set of tentative and somewhat arbitrary clusters. This determination can be made on the basis of intuition, prior knowledge, or, for example, if the investigator feels that there will be six clusters, by stating that the first six objects are the nuclei or seeds of them. The next step is to examine each object and place it in the cluster it most resembles. At this point, most objects have been assigned to one of the groups, and the investigator calculates the centroids of each cluster. Now each object is compared with each centroid, which means that some of the objects may have to be reassigned to different clusters. This necessitates recomputing the centroids and sifting through all the objects yet again. The process of comparison, assignment, and calculation of centroids is repeated, or iterated, until no object needs to be reassigned from one iteration to another.

The various partitioning techniques differ in terms of how the initial clusters are formed, how the final number of clusters are determined, and in the criteria for group membership. We've already discussed the first point briefly, mentioning various options from which the researcher can choose. There are also some empirical methods, such as considering that all of the objects belong to one large heterogeneous group. Then, by some statistical criterion, the group is split into two parts, so that the members of one group are more similar to each other than to the members in the other part.

This splitting process is continued until the optimum number of clusters is reached. This may sound a bit like divisive hierarchical clustering, but there is an important difference: there is no assumption that the two "daughter" groups are subsets of the larger group. In partitioning cluster analysis, once a larger group is divided, it ceases to exist as an entity in its own right.

With some forms of partitioning analysis, the investigator must decide at the outset how many clusters will exist at the end, based again on either prior knowledge or sheer guesswork. Other procedures can add or subtract to this initial estimate, depending on the data. If two clusters get too close together, they are merged; if one cluster becomes too heterogeneous, it is split. As usual, religious wars have sprung up over this. On the one hand, the researcher may not know how many groups to expect, so a more empirical criterion is preferred. On the other hand, though, a nonthinking approach can lead to a solution that doesn't make sense on a clinical basis.

Partitioning methods generally use different criteria for group membership than hierarchical methods use, but the general principles are the same. The two major points of similarity are that (1) each criterion tries to make the groups homogeneous and different from the other clusters and (2) each criterion yields dramatically different results. With so many ways of clustering, computing similarity indices, and determining group membership, it's obviously impossible in one short chapter to go into any depth about the specifics. But any article that uses cluster analytic techniques should spell out in some detail the exact steps used and *why* those, as opposed to some other set of procedures, were used. Consequently, our C.R.A.P. Detectors focus on this point.

C.R.A.P. DETECTORS

C.R.A.P. Detector XVIII-1

Did the authors specify the analytic method used? At the very least, they should state whether they used a hierarchical or a partitioning model although this may be evident from the results. However, it may not be as readily apparent as if they used some other model, or whether an agglomerative or a divisive solution was chosen. The choice of model can produce markedly different results. There should also be some justification for this choice on theoretical grounds.

C.R.A.P. Detector XVIII-2

Was the similarity index specified? Did the authors use a Pearson correlation as their index, followed by a Q-type (or "inverse") factor analysis?

This technique has been supplanted by far superior ones over the past two decades, so if its use has not been well justified, ignore the study.

C.R.A.P. Detector XVIII-3

Did they specify the criterion to determine the number of clusters? Again, this may be fixed by the investigator (and if so, why that number of clusters) or determined on statistical grounds. If the latter, which criterion was used?

C.R.A.P. Detector XVIII-4

Did they state which computer program or algorithm they used? One study found that using exactly the same options with different programs led to different solutions. In order to replicate the results (and see where the other guys went wrong), you should be able to find the program in the computing center or in a specific book.

C.R.A.P. Detector XVIII-5

Did the authors replicate their results? Because so many results with multivariate procedures don't hold up on replication, don't believe the findings until they have been replicated on a different sample and preferably by different authors.

19

Canonical Correlation

Canonical correlation is an extension of multiple regression. Instead of many predictor variables and one dependent variable (DV), there are now multiple DVs.

U*p to this point,* we've dealt with two classes of correlational
statistics: one in which we have just two variables (Pearson's *r* for interval
and ratio data, and Spearman's rho, Kendall's tau, and a few others for ordinal data) and a second in which we have a number of independent variables
(IVs) and one DV (multiple regression). There are situations, though, for
which we would like to explore the *interrelationship between two sets of
variables.*

A major problem all medical schools face is trying to predict who of all
the applicants would make the best physicians 4 years down the road.
Admissions committees look at a variety of preadmission variables such as
university grade point average (GPA), Medical College Admission Test
(MCAT) scores, letters of reference, and so on. Let's assume that a school is
reevaluating its procedures and thus decides to wait a few years and see how
these factors relate to the end product. Because the committee has some
degree of sophistication, it knows that being a good doctor demands more
than just knowledge; it also requires clinical skills. Now let's take a leap of
faith and assume that the school can actually measure these two attributes
with some degree of accuracy. What can the committee members do with
all the data they collect?

There are a number of options available. For example, the committee can
compute two multiple regression equations, regressing the preadmission
variables against each of the outcomes separately. However, this approach
assumes that the outcomes are totally independent of each other, and we can
safely assume that they're not. The equations will be correct, but it will be

difficult to determine the correct probability levels of the statistical tests associated with them. Another alternative would be to combine the two outcome scores into one global measure of performance. This approach has two drawbacks. First, it ignores the **pattern of response**, in that a person high on knowledge and low on clinical skills might have the same global score as a person with the opposite characteristics. The relationship between the two variables may be important, but it will be missed with this method. Second, this approach assumes that knowledge and skills have equal weights (ie, are assumed to be equally important), which may be an unduly limiting restriction. A third method would be to find the best "weights" for the preadmission scores and the best weights for the outcomes that would maximize the correlation between the two sets of variables. This is the approach taken in **canonical correlation**, which we examine in this chapter.

As we've said, canonical correlation can be thought of as an extension of multiple linear regression, but one in which we are predicting to two or more variables instead of just to one. In fact, we even ignore the distinction between "dependent" and "independent" variables and think of canonical correlation as a method of exploring the relationship between two sets of variables. One set can be called the "predictors" and the other called the "criteria," or we can do away with these labels entirely. For example, set 1 can consist of scores on a test battery at time 1, and set 2 can comprise scores from the same test administered at a later time. This would be the multivariate analogue of test-retest reliability, where our interest is not in prediction but in the temporal stability of results. In a different situation, we may gather a number of measures regarding the physical status of cancer patients and a second set of scores on their psychological status. Again, our concern is not in predicting physical status from mental status or vice versa, but rather, in seeing if any relationship exists between these two sets of scores.

CANONICAL VARIATES AND VARIABLES

Let's review what we have so far. Our research has gathered two sets of variables: set A, consisting of three preadmission scores, and set B, consisting of two performance indices. The first step in canonical correlation would be to derive two **canonical variates**, one for each set of scores. These are not some sort of religious heretics but are simply scores based on the variables in each set. For example, if x_1 is the score for GPA, x_2 the MCAT score, and x_3 the score for the letters of reference, then:

$$x_A = B_1x_1 + B_2x_2 + B_3x_3$$

Put into English, the canonical variate for set A (which we've designated x_A) is derived by multiplying each variable by some "beta weight."

In a similar manner, we compute a canonical variate for the variables in set B (consisting of variables x_5 and x_6), which we'll call x_B. Just to reinforce some of the jargon we'll be using later, "variables" refers to our original measures (GPA, MCAT, and so on) while "variates" refers to our derived scores, based on multiplying each variable by some weighting factor. The two sets of beta weights (one for set A and one for set B) are chosen to maximize the correlation between x_A and x_B. How this is done is beyond the scope of this book; suffice it to say that no other combination of weights will yield a higher correlation.

PARTIAL CORRELATION

The beta weights are, in essence, **partial correlations**. We'll briefly review what this means because it has major implications for what follows. If we have two predictor variables, such as age (A) and serum cholesterol (B), and one criterion variable, such as degree of stenosis (Y), then we can compute simple run-of-the-mill correlations between each of the predictors and the criterion. Let's make up some figures and assume r_{AY} is 0.75 and r_{BY} is 0.70. But we know that age and cholesterol are themselves correlated, say, at the 0.65 level. Then, the partial correlation between B and Y is the correlation *after removing the contribution of age* to both cholesterol and stenosis. In this case, the figure drops from 0.70 to 0.42.

So, the beta weight for variable x_1 is the correlation between x_1 and x_A, eliminating the effects of x_2 and x_3; the beta weight for x_2 eliminates x_1 and x_3, and so forth.

What this means for canonical correlation is that the two canonical variates that we've derived, x_A and x_B, do not account for all of the variance since only that portion of the variance *uncorrelated with the other variables in the set* was used. We can extract another pair of canonical variates that accounts for at least some of the remaining variability. How many pairs of equations can we get? If we have n variables in set A and m variables in set B, then the number of canonical correlations is the smaller of the two numbers. In our example, n is 3 and m is 2, so there will be two canonical correlations, or two pairs of canonical variates, x_{A1} paired with x_{B1} and x_{A2} paired with x_{B2}.

In some ways, these variates are similar to the factors in exploratory factor analysis. First, they are extracted in order, so that the first one accounts for more of the variance than the second, the second more than the third (if we had a third one), and so on. Second, they are uncorrelated with each other ("orthogonal," to use the jargon). Third, not all of them need to be statistically significant. We usually hope that at least the first one is, but we may reach a point where one pair of variates, and all of the succeeding ones, may not be. There is a statistical test, based on the chi-square, that can tell us how many of the correlations are significant, in fact.

REDUNDANCY

So, what we need at this point are two types of significance tests. First, we have to check how many (if any) of the canonical correlations are significant. As we already mentioned, this is done by a chi-square test developed by Bartlett. Second, if at least one correlation (R_c) is significant, then we have to see if the variables in one set account for a significant proportion of the variance in the other set's variables.

One measure of this is called **redundancy**, which tries to do for canonical correlation what r^2 does for the Pearson correlation. However, unlike r^2, redundancy is not symmetrical; that is, if r^2 is 0.39, then 39% of the variance of variable X can be explained by variable Y, and 39% of the variance of Y can be accounted for by X. But, in the multivariate case, set A may account for 50% of the variance in the set B variables, but set B may account for only 30% of the set A variance. The figures for redundancy are always less than the square of R_c; they are often much less and may be as low as 10%, even if the magnitude of R_c is quite respectable.

STATISTICAL SIGNIFICANCE

For our original example, the first table that we would see from a computer printout would look something like Table 19-1. The table is not really as formidable as it first appears. The eigenvalue is simply the square of the canonical correlation and is interpreted in the same way as R^2 in multiple regression: the first set of canonical variates shares 73% of their variance, and the second set shares 55%. Lambda is a measure of the significance of the correlation, and as always, the smaller values are more significant. Through a bit of statistical hand waving, lambda is transformed into Bartlett's chi-square, which humans (ie, nonstatisticians) find easier to interpret. This table tells us that both equations are statistically significant.

Table 19-1

Significance of Two Canonical Correlations

Number	Eigenvalue	Canonical Correlation	Wilks' Lambda	Chi-square	D.F.	Significance
1	0.732	0.856	0.121	202.953	6	< 0.001
2	0.549	0.741	0.451	76.450	2	< 0.001

Table 19-2

Beta Weights for the Two Equations

	Set 1			Set 2	
	V1	**V2**	**V3**	**V4**	**V5**
Equation 1	0.803	0.657	0.260	0.960	0.259
Equation 2	−0.115	−0.182	0.966	−0.279	0.966

Having found at least one equation significant, the next step is to figure out the pattern of the variables. What we would then look for in a computer printout would resemble Table 19-2. Notice that this simulated output labels the variables as V1 through V5; others may use X's or the variable names.

We would interpret this as meaning that there are two patterns of responding. People who have high GPAs (V1) and high MCAT scores (V2) do well on knowledge-based criteria (V4). Students who did well in clinical skills (V5) were those with good letters of reference (V3). Most of the time, the results are not nearly as clear-cut, but the general principles remain the same.

Although the canonical correlations and eigenvalues were quite high, we cannot assume that redundancy is also high. Actually, there are four redundancies here: how much of the variance the set 1 variables explain of set 2 for equation 1 (r_{11}) and for equation 2 (r_{12}) and how much the set 2 variables explain of set 1 for equations 1 (r_{21}) and 2 (r_{22}).

The calculations are really quite simple, being the Sum of Squares of each coefficient divided by the number of coefficients, times the eigenvalue. For r_{11}, this would be:

$$[(0.803)^2 + (0.657)^2 + (0.260)^2]/N \times 0.732 = 0.279$$

Just for the sake of completeness, $r_{12} = 0.362$, $r_{21} = 0.179$, and $r_{22} = 0.278$. These, then, tell a somewhat different story, with much of the variance awaiting to be explained.

C.R.A.P. DETECTORS

C.R.A.P. Detector XIX-1

What was the ratio of subjects to variables? This issue rears its ugly head yet again. As before, there should be at least 10 subjects for each variable, and some authors recommend a 30:1 ratio. Even if we split the difference, we can ignore most articles because they don't come even close to a 20:1 ratio.

C.R.A.P. Detector XIX-2

Are the R_c values significant? If this important statistic was not mentioned, read no further. However, as we've discussed, don't let the reporters get away with reporting *only* the significance level of R_c; there's more yet to come.

C.R.A.P. Detector XIX-3

Do they report redundancy? Actually, they need not report redundancy per se, but there should be some estimate of the variance in one set attributable to the other set. The actual statistic may be a predictive one or some other one, but it must be mentioned somewhere.

C.R.A.P. Detector XIX-4

Was the study cross-validated? As we've said before, multivariate statistics always look good on the original sample. However, don't trust the results unless they've been cross-validated on a new sample or on a hold-out sample (ie, deriving the equations on about 75% of the original sample and testing its "goodness" on the remaining 25%).

20

Reprise

> In this section, we discuss various ways you can present data graphically (and a few ways you shouldn't) and how to solve some of the problems of dealing with missing data.

GRAPHING

While reading this book, you've come across different types of graphs. Some have vertical bars while others use continuous lines; some use smooth curves, and others look like flights of stairs. In this section, we'll explain the rationale behind the choices and why certain graphs do *not* sully these august pages. To begin, though, we'll explain what we should expect graphs to do and what they shouldn't be asked to do.

Most important, graphs are not tables. When we draw a graph, we expect the reader to almost intuitively grasp the *relationship* between variables—that category *A* is more prevalent than *C* and that *B* is endorsed least; or that as variable *X* increases, *Y* decreases; or that people improve faster with one form of therapy than another. The actual magnitudes of the variables are of secondary interest at best. If you want your readers to know that exactly 29.38% of psoriasis sufferers got better with clam juice and that 32.57% got better with chicken soup, use a table; don't expect that these precise numbers will be apparent from a graph. At the same time, don't go messing up your graph by sticking numbers inside of it. A second point is that, with few exceptions, less is better. Determine what message you want to get across (note the deliberate use of the singular), and cut out everything else; that's why all graphing packages have a little scissors on top—to expurgate junk.

Bar Charts, Histograms, and Line Charts

Bar charts are just what their name says they are: bars that represent the amounts (frequency, percent, or magnitude) in various categories. For example, we can show the data from Table 5-1—the mean pain ratings of people taking various acetylsalicylic acid (ASA) compounds—by using a bar graph, as in Figure 20-1. It takes a bit more work to determine the actual values (and this would be even more so with real data that weren't whole numbers), but the relative effectiveness of the different brands is much more obvious than they were in the table.

We can make the graph even more informative by recognizing that group is a nominal variable; that is, the alphabetical ordering is completely arbitrary. We don't lose any information if we shuffle the order; in fact, by rank-ordering the groups as in Figure 20-2, we make the relationships easier to see. We can't do this with ordinal data, as would be the case if each group had an increasing amount of the active agent or if we were plotting the number of people falling into the categories of Fail, Below Average, Average, Above Average, and Excellent. In these cases, the order is meaningful, and we would actually make the graph more difficult to understand by rearranging the categories.

There's one subtle point about bar charts: there's a gap between the bars. This isn't mere aesthetics; it reflects the fact that the categories are distinct and separate from one another. When we graph continuous data, such as height, blood pressure, serum rhubarb, intelligence quotient (IQ), or what-

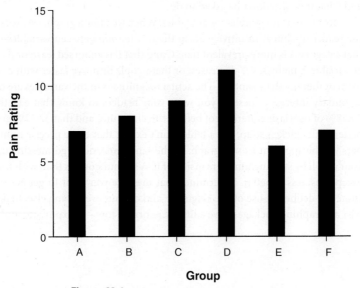

Figure 20-1 A simple bar chart of the data in Table 5-1.

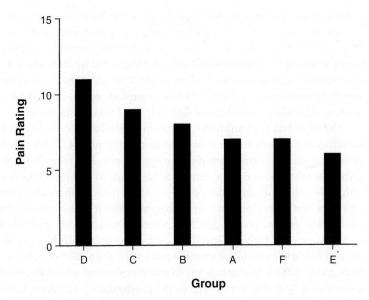

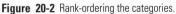

Figure 20-2 Rank-ordering the categories.

ever, the bars abut one another. In honor of this change in appearance, we give this type of graph a new name: **histogram**. In Figure 20-3, we've plotted the number of E-mail messages marked "urgent" sent each day by 100 hospital administrators. Note that the bars are touching or nearly touching.

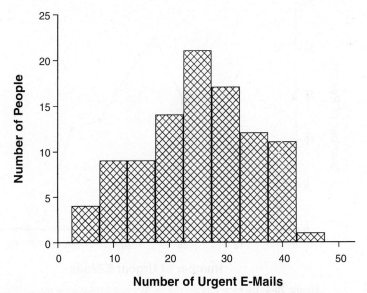

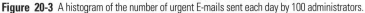

Figure 20-3 A histogram of the number of urgent E-mails sent each day by 100 administrators.

In this case, each bar represents a range of values. The first bar, with the value 5, covers the range from 3 to 7; the one labeled 10 spans 8 to 12; and so on. This means that we've lost some information. We know that there were four people who sent between three and seven messages, but we don't know the exact number sent by each of the four people. The wider the interval, the more information we lose. Later, we'll look at one technique—stem-and-leaf plotting—that allows us to both make a graph and preserve the data.

When the data are continuous, we can forgo the bars and simply draw a continuous line from the center of each bar, as in Figure 20-4. This is called, for obvious reasons, a **line chart**. If you compare Figure 20-4 with Figure 20-3, you'll see that the line was extended at both ends so that it touches 0 at both ends—again, a convention, more for looks than anything else. One advantage that a line chart has over histograms is that it's easier to compare two or three groups, as in Figure 20-5, where we've added the number of such messages sent by clinicians. If the data were displayed as histograms, our eyes would allow us to compare the groups at a given value of X, but it's much more difficult to compare the overall distributions when compared to line charts. Note that, in this case, we didn't extend the graph down to the x-axis on the left side, because that would have resulted in a meaningless number, one that was less than 0. This reinforces the point that conventions are fine but that they shouldn't interfere with common sense.

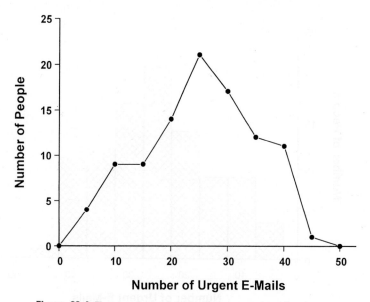

Figure 20-4 The same data as in Figure 20-3, presented as a line chart.

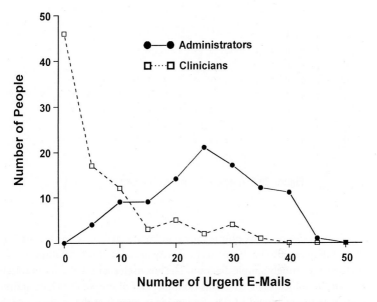

Figure 20-5 Displaying two groups in a line chart.

Stem-and-Leaf Plots and Box Plots

Over the past 20 years or so, two new ways of displaying data have become more popular: stem-and-leaf plots and box plots, both from the fertile mind of John Tukey. **Stem-and-leaf plots** allow us to display the data as a histogram without losing any information caused by putting a range of values into a single bar. If you turn Figure 20-6 on its side (or leave it as is and look at it while lying down), you'll see that it has the same shape as Figure 20-3, which is gratifying, because it's showing the same data. The left-most column is the number of subjects in that line. The next column is called the **stem** and contains the digits that are most significant. Our data go from 4 to 47, so if we were to use one row for every decade (0–9, 10–19, etc), there would be only five rows. Aesthetically, it would be better to have somewhere between 7 and 15 rows, so we split each decade in half. Consequently, the first 0 in that column is for the numbers 0 to 4, and the second 0 is for the numbers 5 to 9; the first 1 (row 3) is for the numbers 10 to 14, and the second 1 is for the numbers 15 to 19; and so on.

The remaining numbers in each row are the **leaves**, and they are the less significant digits. So if we look at the third row, where the stem is 1 and the leaves are 0 0 1 1 2 2 3 4 4, we'd know there were two people who sent 10 urgent E-mails, two who sent 11, two who sent 12, one who sent 13, and two who sent 14—an elegant way of having our cake and eating it, too.

x

0	0:
4	0: 5 5 7 9
9	1: 0 0 1 1 2 2 3 4 4
9	1: 5 6 6 7 7 8 9 9 9
14	2: 0 0 0 1 1 1 1 2 2 2 3 4 4 4
21	2: 5 5 5 5 6 6 6 7 7 7 7 7 7 7 8 8 8 9 9 9
17	3: 0 0 0 0 1 1 2 2 2 3 3 3 3 4 4 4 4
12	3: 5 5 6 6 6 6 7 7 8 8 9 9
11	4: 0 1 1 1 2 2 2 2 3 3 4
1	4: 7

Figure 20-6 A stem-and-leaf plot of the data in Figure 20-4.

An example of a **box plot** is shown in Figure 20-7; this one is horizontal, but they can also be drawn vertically. Again, a lot of information is conveyed in a seemingly simple diagram. The box itself spans the range in which 50% of the subjects fall, so in this example, half of the subjects have scores that are between 10 and 34. The line inside the box is at the median, which is about 18 in this case. Furthermore, 95% of the cases fall within the range defined by "whiskers" with short bars at each end (3 and 42), which define the *inner fences*. In this example, there is one *outlier*, whose score is greater than the inner fences but less than the (undrawn) *outer fences*, which encompass 98% of the subjects. Finally, there are two *extreme outliers*, whose scores are in the upper or lower 1%. Some computer programs actually print the case numbers of the outliers and extreme outliers, so it's easy to determine

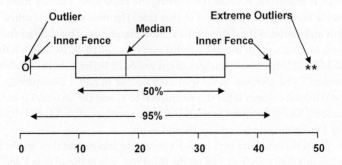

Figure 20-7 The gross anatomy of a box plot.

whether they really have extreme scores or whether someone made an error while entering the data. As a final wrinkle, we can make the width of the box proportional to the sample size. This is handy when two or more box plots are drawn next to one another; we can see how much the groups differ in size, and we can temper our interpretations in light of that.

How *Not* to Draw Graphs

Actually, the best places to get examples of graphs that should never have seen the light of day are newspapers (especially if they have a horoscope column, and most of all, if they also have a full-page weather map in color) and at presentations made to impress administrators. We're not as creative as Moses, so we'll present only four commandments.

First, *Thou shalt not make thy bars look three-dimensional.* They look sexy as all get-out, but it's difficult to see where the top is as we're often deceived by the back edge of the bar. This is particularly true if the *y*-axis also looks three-dimensional because we have to mentally extend the top of the box to the axis and then look down at an angle to read off the value. The more extreme the three-dimensional look, the worse the problem is. As if this isn't bad enough, one very popular program makes things infinitely worse by using the *back* of the box to indicate the magnitude whereas we expect the front to be the value.

Second, *Thou shalt honor the bar and keep it holy.* Displaying the number of people in each group by stacking up little people icons is cutesy, as is showing costs with piles of coins or dollar signs. Avoid the temptation; it's nothing but "chart junk" that should be exiled into the wilderness, yea verily, and declared outcast and anathema.

Third, *Thou shalt not commit a stacked bar graph.* An example of this abomination is shown in Figure 20-8. We can easily compare the relative number of single people across groups because they all have a common baseline. But are there more divorced people in Group B or Group C? That's much more difficult. We have to mentally shift the box in Group C down until the bottom lines up with Group B, keeping the height constant as we move it. It's not difficult; it's darned near impossible.

Fourth, *Thou shalt not suffer multiple pie charts to grace thy pages.* Pie charts aren't so bad if we're displaying the data for just one group, but they're useless for comparing groups. It's the same problem as with stacked bar graphs. We can compare the first wedge across groups because all first wedges start at the 12:00 position. After that, though, we have to mentally rotate the wedge from one group to make it line up with that from the other group in order to compare angles. Again, try to compare the proportions of divorced people in Figure 20-9. Now imagine the task if we drew pies for all five groups. If you have to put in numbers to make the pie charts understandable, then

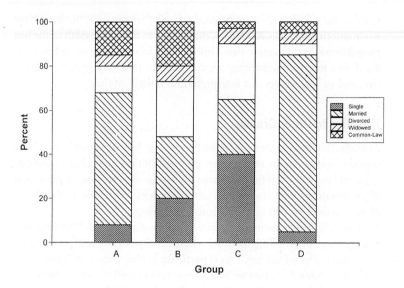

Figure 20-8 A stacked box plot.

either use a table or a different type of graph. Remember, the only time a pie chart is appropriate is at a baker's convention.

DEALING WITH MISSING DATA

Open up any statistics book (including this one, so far) and you'll find beautiful tables of data to be analyzed. If the text describes a *t* test with 10 subjects in each group, there are the 20 numbers just waiting to be summed and squared and added; if the next chapter has a repeated measures analysis of

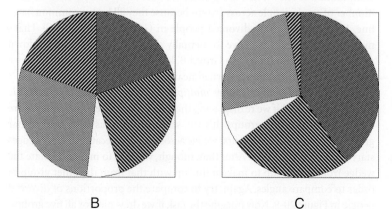

Figure 20-9 A pie chart.

variance (ANOVA) with five testing periods, then the numbers are nicely lined up, all in their proper place. This may reflect the situation in some psychology experiments. For example, if a rat shucks its mortal coil in the midst of an experiment, it's replaced with the next one in the cage; or if a student doesn't show up for the study, he or she is replaced (and often given demerit points, but that's a separate story). In the real world, though, life isn't so straightforward. If people refuse to be interviewed or if patients drop out of a trial of a new intervention, we can't simply replace them and pretend that nothing has happened. First of all, we may not be able to replace a participant, because of time or budgetary constraints or because the pool of eligible patients is limited. More important, though, most applied researchers believe in the dictum that people do not drop out of studies for trivial reasons. They may stop coming for follow-up visits because (1) they got better and don't see the need to waste their time filling out questionnaires or having blood drawn, (2) they didn't get better and are off looking for someone who can help them, (3) they find the side effects of the treatment too burdensome, or (4) they may have succumbed to the effects of the therapy or the lack of therapy. Some people may stop participating because of factors unrelated to the treatment, such as finding a job in a new town, but for the most part, the reasons for the loss of data are related to the treatment itself. If we replace the participant with someone who stays in the study, then we may be biasing the results by eliminating from the analysis people with positive or negative outcomes. The bottom line is that we have to find some way of dealing with the missing data. In this section, we'll discuss some of the ways that have been developed to work around the problems.

Ignoring the Missing Data

A purist would say that we don't know the values of the missing data and that any attempt to *impute* them (ie, make up a value) belongs on the shelf marked "Fiction" rather than that marked "Truth and Beauty." Strictly speaking, they're right; if there are relatively few missing data points (roughly 5% of the values), ignoring them is probably the safest thing to do. The difficulty is that the effects of missing data can multiply rapidly. When the variables with the missing data are used in multivariable procedures such as multiple regression or factor analysis, most computer programs rightly use what's called *listwise deletion*, omitting the subject (with all of his or her data) from the analysis. If there are five variables and each is missing 5% of the values at random, then it's possible that up to 25% of the subjects will be eliminated, which can seriously jeopardize the results. So if up to 5% of the values of a variable are missing and if that variable won't be combined with any others (eg, you're just using "age" to describe the sample, not as a predictor variable), just live with it. But if more values are missing or if the variable will be combined with others, you'll have to find some other ways of handling the situation.

Replacing with the Mean

Replacing a missing value with the group's mean value will, by definition, not change the mean at all. For this reason, as well as the fact that it's easy to do, many people opt for this approach. But there's a drawback. Because it's highly unlikely that all of the missing values were in fact equal to the mean, the result is that we've reduced the standard deviation (SD) of that variable. By making the SD smaller, we also make the standard error (SE) smaller, and since the SE goes into the denominator of most statistical tests, we've artificially inflated the probability of finding a difference between groups.

Hot-Deck Imputation

A step up in sophistication, hot-deck imputation involves finding a similar person among the subjects and using that person's score. For example, let's say one person refused to enter her age (yes, we're being sexist; so what else is new?). We would look for a woman who was similar to her on one or two other variables (ideally, some that are correlated with age) and use this person's age as the value for the person with the missing data. If there are a number of such people (as we hope there are), one is selected at random. This results in a more accurate estimate of the score because the value is realistic and includes some degree of measurement error. The downside of this approach is that it reduces the estimate of the SD. It also requires a large sample size in order to find people with similar scores, which is why we find that this technique is used mainly in large epidemiologic studies.

Multiple Regression

However, why use just a few people to impute the missing value? If age is related to some other variables in the data set, we can use all the people and run a multiple regression with age as the dependent variable and those other variables as predictors. This is easier to do, and it doesn't require us to find people who are similar on a number of factors, making it more feasible. In fact, this is the approach used by many statistical software packages. However, it has the same drawback as replacing with the mean, in that it results in a reduced estimate of the SD. We can get around this by using the value predicted by the regression equation and then adding a "fudge factor," which is some error based on the SD of the predicted values. This means that if two people have the same predicted scores, they will each get somewhat different imputed scores. Because of this, we preserve the SD of the variable.

It requires a bit more work, but we are repaid, in that the resulting statistical tests aren't quite as biased as they would otherwise be.

Last Observation Carried Forward

Last observation carried forward (LOCF) is probably the most widely used technique in drug trials and has gained the seal of approval from the Food and Drug Administration. The name says it all; when a person drops out of a study, the last recorded value is "carried forward" to fill in the blanks. The logic is that this is conservative, operating against the hypothesis that people will get better over time, and so it supposedly underestimates the degree of improvement. The advantages of LOCF are that it is easy to do and that we do not lose subjects. However, there are some problems with this technique. The first is the assumption that no change occurs aside from the effect of the intervention. This may indeed be a conservative assumption for the experimental group but is actually quite liberal with regard to the control or comparison group. It ignores the fact that the natural history of many disorders, ranging from depression to lower back pain, is improvement over time, even in the absence of treatment. This is especially true if the person is on a comparator drug or intervention rather than placebo. The newer nonsteroidal anti-inflammatories, for example, are no more effective than the older ones; their purported advantage is in the side effect profile. Consequently, patients may drop out of the arm with the older agents not because they aren't improving but because they are having problems with an upset stomach. The assumption that they will not continue to improve may underestimate the efficacy of these drugs. So when applied to the control group, LOCF may artificially inflate the difference between the groups, in favor of the experimental one.

The second problem is that when LOCF is used with negative outcomes, such as adverse drug reactions, it underestimates their consequences by assuming that they will not get worse over time. The third problem, which is related to the first two, is that LOCF ignores all of the data points before the last one; that is, LOCF doesn't make use of the "trajectory" of how the subject was improving or getting worse.

Multiple Imputation

The state of the art (at least as of last Tuesday) is a technique called *multiple imputation*. We won't even try to explain the math, because it makes our brains want to shrivel up and die. To keep it simple, multiple imputation uses regression-like statistics many times, with different starting values each time. The final imputed value for each missing data point is the mean of these estimates. The real advantage comes from the fact that it estimates not only the mean, but based on how much the guesses differ from each other, it can build in the variability that is present in the data. The end result is that the final data set, with the imputed values, gives unbiased estimates of means, variances, and other parameters. Amazingly, this technique comes up with fairly accurate estimates even when up to 20% of the data are missing for a single variable.

Research Designs

21

As we $mentioned$ in the Introduction, statistical methods are excellent for dealing with random variation, but they're not too useful for eliminating bias in experiments, which must be approached by using appropriate experimental designs. Below is a description of several of the more common research designs. Many others exist, and those who are interested should consult one or more of the books listed in the Bibliography.

TYPES OF RESEARCH DESIGNS

Randomized Control Trial

The randomized control trial (RCT) provides the strongest research design. A group of people are *randomly* allocated by the researcher to two or more groups. The experimental group receives the new treatment whereas the control group receives either conventional therapy, a placebo, or nothing. For example, our psoriasis patients would be split into two groups by the flip of a coin. The "heads" group would receive clam juice, and the "tails" group would receive a placebo concoction. Ideally, in order to minimize various biases, neither the patient nor the researcher knows who got what until the trial is over. This is referred to as being "double blind." (If the pharmacist who dispensed the stuff loses the code, it can be called either a "triple blind" or a disaster. In either case, the pharmacist's life is in jeopardy.) More than two groups can be used in an RCT as long as subjects are allocated by some randomizing device.

The major advantage of the RCT is that it ensures that there are no systematic differences between the groups. Because they originally are drawn at random from the same population, randomization ensures that they will be identical except for the differences that might arise from chance. In fact, the basis of many statistical tests of hypotheses is that the groups are drawn randomly from a population.

However, there are two major drawbacks to the RCT. The first is the cost. Some of the trials designed to look at the effect of aspirin on re-infarction rate cost between $3 and $7 million, and the most expensive one of all (at least until now), which was designed to look at lipids and infarction, costs $150 million US! The second major drawback is that patients who volunteer to participate in an RCT and who agree to allow the management of their disease to be decided by the flip of a coin may not be representative of patients in general.

Cohort Study

One alternative to the RCT is the cohort study. In this type of study, two groups (or "cohorts") of subjects are identified: one that by choice, luck, or chance has been exposed to the clinical intervention or putative causal agent, and one that has not been exposed. Our researcher, for example, can try to locate a group of clam juice drinkers and compare the proportion of those who have psoriasis in that group with the porportion of those with psoriasis in a group of abstainers.

Although good cohort studies are not cheap, they are often less expensive than RCTs because the groups are preexisting, and the elaborate safeguards necessary to follow cases prospectively for several years are unnecessary. However, their primary advantages may be feasibility and ethics. If we're studying a helpful intervention, it is not being withheld from those who want it or being given to those who don't. Further, it is patently unethical to deliberately expose people to a potentially harmful agent (such as tobacco smoke or asbestos fibers), so research on health risks must inevitably use this approach. In a cohort study, we locate a group of people who have chosen to smoke or who have been in contact with the putative cause owing to their work, place of residence, travel, or whatever, and thereby avoid these ethical issues.

The major disadvantage is that it is impossible to be sure that the groups are comparable in terms of other factors that may influence the results. For example, smoking is related to social class, and jobs that involve exposure to carcinogens are usually related to social class as well. So if smokers have a higher incidence of lung cancer than nonsmokers, is it attributable to smoking, social class, occupational exposure, or something else? Even with carefully selected controls, we can never be sure. A second drawback is that if a certain treatment has become popular for a disorder (eg, anxiolytics for phobias), it may be hard to find untreated controls. A third drawback is that it is difficult, if not impossible, to maintain "blindness," at least in the subjects.

Prospective Survey

The prospective survey is similar to the cohort study, but only one group is chosen initially. Some of the subjects will become exposed to the intervention or putative causal agent over time, and others will not. Therefore, the outcomes can be observed in these naturally occurring groups some time down the road.

The advantages and disadvantages are similar to those of the cohort study, but there are some additional disadvantages, the primary one being that at the end, there may be too few subjects in one group to allow for proper analyses.

Case-Control Study

In a case-control study, a group of people who already have the outcome (cases) is matched with a group who do not (controls), and the researcher determines the proportion in each who had previously been exposed to the suspected causal factor. For instance, in one study, the use of exogenous estrogens in one group of women with endometrial cancer was compared to that in a disease-free control group. The researchers found that more of the cancer patients reported using the hormone than did subjects in the other group. However, the weakness of this method was pointed out by a later study, which took as its starting point the supposition that estrogens do not cause cancer but do lead to bleeding. These women came to the attention of physicians because of the bleeding, who then performed biopsies to discover the cause and found cancer. Women who did not experience bleeding may have had the same incidence of endometrial cancer as those who did, but since no biopsies were performed on them, they were never diagnosed. When using controls to account for this, these researchers found a much lower risk of cancer attributable to estrogens. Because the design was retrospective, it could not account for other factors that could lead to the outcome. However, in circumstances in which the outcome is rare or the time from exposure to outcome is long, this may be the only feasible approach. For example, in most studies of occupational risks related to cancer, in which relatively few people actually go on to develop the disease, delays of 10 to 20 years may be involved.

Cross-Sectional Survey

An even weaker method of establishing causal relationships than the prospective survey or the case-control study is the cross-sectional design, which also uses one group. At one point in time, the subjects are interviewed and/or examined to determine whether or not they were exposed to the agent and whether they have the outcome of interest. For example, a large group of women could be interviewed to determine (1) if they had given birth to a child with a cleft lip and (2) if they had used tricyclic antidepressants during the pregnancy. A higher proportion of women who used these medications and had children with this deformity may indicate that the antidepressant was responsible.

Cross-sectional surveys are relatively cheap, and subjects neither are deliberately exposed to possibly harmful agents nor have treatments withheld from them or imposed on them. However, in addition to having all the problems of prospective surveys, cross-sectional designs have another major problem in that it may not be possible to state what is cause and what is effect. Schizophrenics, for instance, have larger cerebral ventricles than nonschizophrenics, thus raising the question of whether the enlarged ventricles are responsible for the schizophrenia or are a result of it (in fact, they may be caused by the neuroleptic medication).

Before–After Design

In a before–after research design, the outcome is assessed before and after some intervention in one group of subjects. Although common, this design is also weak because the change may be attributable to some other factor. For example, the fact that a group of nursing students scores higher on a multiple-choice test after a course in geriatrics than before does not allow the teacher to take credit for their increased knowledge. They may have taken an elective at a nursing home or made a visit to Grandma's house, or they may have benefited from taking the examination the first time. Worse still, differences based on a single measure, before and after, may not reflect any intervention at all, just maturation over time.

To some degree, these problems can be dealt with by taking multiple measures as described in Chapter 9, "Time Series Analysis," but the possibility that something else happened co-incident in time with the treatment cannot be excluded.

IMPLICATIONS FOR STATISTICS

What do all these different designs (and there are many others we haven't touched on) have to do with statistics? Both quite a bit and not too much, at the same time. For the most part, the decision to use either one or another statistical test depends on the measure more than on the design. The results of an RCT can be analyzed with a chi-square or a similar test if the outcome of interest is normal or ordinal, such as death or degree of functional improvement as measured on a three-point scale. By the same token, t tests or analyses of variance (ANOVAs) could be used for continuous outcomes such as blood pressure; multivariate analysis of variance (MANOVA) for multiple dependent measures; life table analyses, for length of survival; and so on. Similarly, the outcome of a prospective or case-control study could be looked at by comparing the proportion of survivors and nonsurvivors in various groups or by correlating the amount of the outcome (such as a measure of lung function) with some other factor (such as the number of cigarettes smoked or the length of time at a smelter). So the choice of statistical test is not really related to the experimental design.

However, the statistical tests of significance are predicated on the supposition that the samples were drawn at random from the population. This assumption is violated to a greater or lesser degree in most designs other than the RCT, so that the results in such designs have to be interpreted with some caution, both in terms of the actual significance level and in terms of inferring that the results are attributable to the experimental variable and not something else.

Index